Fredericka Charles

——BATTLING——
Eczema & Allergies

Diary of a Desperate Mother

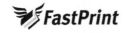

www.fast-print.net/store.php

Diary of a Desperate Mother
©Fredericka Charles 2014
www.diaryofadesperatemother.com

A catalogue record for this book is available from the British Library

ISBN 978-178456-053-9

Cover design & layout by David Springer

First published 2014 by
FASTPRINT PUBLISHING
Peterborough, England.

An environmentally friendly book printed and bound in England by
www.printondemand-worldwide.com

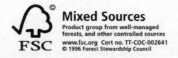

PEFC Certified

This product is
from sustainably
managed forests
and controlled
sources

www.pefc.org

PEFC/16-33-415

8th January 2015

Dear Caroline.

Thank you for your support.
All good things to you

Love Fredericka x

Dedication

To my son Jayden Jean-Paul-Denis, my inspiration.
Without you this would never be.

To you Lord, for giving me the strength to make it through.

To my dear father James Maurice Charles
(1922 – 2013) I dedicate the drive
I have, all to you.

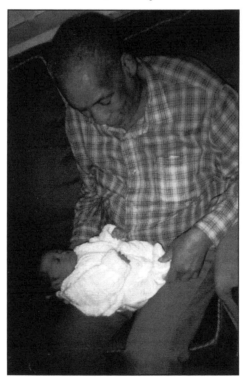

©Fredericka Charles   November 2011

Contents

Acknowledgements

Firstly, I thank God for my very special son, Jayden. I thank you Jayden for being a Champion, for your bravery, endurance and love – without you none of this would have been possible.

I thank God for giving me life and the strength to endure and embrace the journey I have been on.

To Robert Stevenson, from Applejacks, Health Food Shop in East London. Thank you for being my friend and shoulder to cry on, literally. When I felt broken I could run to you and you picked me up every time.

To Bishop Wayne Malcolm, thank you for inspiring and teaching me how to, at long last, give birth to my first book.

To my Editors, Ingrid Charles and Mildred Talabi, I thank you for being as excited as I was about my book, for seeing the vision I hadn't even voiced, running with me and pushing me to get this done.

To my friend and mentor Len Allen thank you, thank you, thank you for being so excellent at what you do and helping me to get back on track when all around me seemed to be collapsing.   Thank you to Karen Allen for helping me to 'Dare to Dream'.

To Sara Coffi, who believed in me from the very beginning, as we waited for our children who acted in 'The Lion King', at London's Lyceum Theatre. Sara would sometimes sit with me in The Strand Palace Hotel in London and, it was there, in September 2010 that I started writing this book in earnest. To the staff and management at the hotel thank you for the welcome and allowing me to write in the comfort of your lounge.

To the NHS, and all the Health Practitioners who helped us along our journey.

To dear Pastor David Springer, Graphic Designer extraordinaire! Thank you for your tireless support, your expertise in making my book look amazing and your patience. You made it all right. You are an excellent man x

Thank you Cyril Peter, Photographer for the people.

To my dear sister Ingrid and the rest of my family, I thank you for giving me all the support I allowed. A special thank you to my friends, Noel Serrano, Alistair Siddon and Joseph Carr, for helping me to shape my book.

Vonnie Hendricks, thank you for keeping the wind beneath my wings. I thank you all for your encouragement and help as I worked towards my dream to write this book and get through my personal battles, thank you from the bottom of my heart.

To my late father James Maurice Charles thank you, I salute you for the quiet wisdom you have imparted in me.

I love you all x

About the Author

Raised in Hackney, London of Dominican parents, Fredericka Charles started her journey in the world of work as a Personal Assistant and part-time model.

Being naturally curious, Fredericka saved hard to see the world and it was whilst visiting foreign countries she realised where her career passion lay ... Health and Fitness. In 1996, Fredericka enrolled at the University of East London where she gained a BA Honours in Health and Fitness. Since then she has worked in a number of Health and Fitness-related roles: in sports clubs as a Fitness Instructor and Duty Manager, on board a cruise liner as the Fitness Director, in Secondary Schools as a Physical Education Teacher and self employed as a Personal Trainer for almost 20 years. She now hosts workshops inspiring people to be the best they can be.

Fredericka's expert skills and patience were needed when her son, Jayden quickly developed severe Eczema and Allergies. Having already studied nutrition at a basic level, Jayden's arrival and subsequent medical conditions further increased

Fredericka's interest in nutrition and paved the way for her to focus her ongoing personal studies on the effects food can have on the body.

Her drive and determination have been instrumental in giving her the knowledge and insight to pen this book and strive to be the best she can be.

Preface

"More people then ever have Eczema as the number of people suffering has almost trebled in 30 years and today 1 in 5 children have the condition. It's a chronic condition that can't be cured but can be managed with attention to diet, environment, skin care and life style". www.MolnlyckeHealthCare.com

Severe Eczema is difficult to treat, it causes a great amount of stress, not only for the sufferer, but for the parents, family and carers. However, my belief is that because many people see it as just 'really dry skin that just needs moisturising' (which is what I believed before I became the mother of a sufferer). It is often overlooked and not given the necessary support and attention it requires, physiologically or psychologically from Health Professionals.

There are plenty of conventional and alternative treatments available, however, sufferers and carers can still feel very alone and confused by the condition as treatment is more often than not, not a cure.

Eczema can be triggered by many different factors, so it is often difficult to establish what the cause is. Even if you manage to establish the cause, and find a remedy for it, reactions to remedies can continuously change. Sometimes a successful treatment today can cease to be effective after a short period of time.

Meeting and talking to someone who is in the same situation as you, can be a powerful tool. You can discuss which treatments work for you and which don't – sometimes the simplest tips are the most effective, even if only for a short time. I met a woman at a health shop who shared with me the importance of using good quality, balanced water to bathe the sufferer. She recommended mineral water. It made sense so I tried it, it made my son more comfortable.

It was not unusual that my son had both Allergies and Eczema as they are in the same family of disease, also included in this are Hay Fever and Asthma. Thank God my son didn't have those to contend with as well. If you or anyone close to you has Eczema and Allergies, you will know how disruptive and difficult they can make life.

The aim of this book is not to give you detailed descriptions of what Eczema or Allergies are, you can find thousands of those online, in the library, in medical journals etc, but it's simply to take you with us as we learned to live with these conditions. Eczema is a disease which leaves the sufferers skin, dry, inflamed, itchy, oozing, red, hot, burning, leathery, rough, scaly, sensitive, crusting, cracked open and bleeding. I'm sure there are many more adjectives but these are what my son experienced.

Food allergies throw the body into extreme responses as it prepares to defend itself from something it has come to know as dangerous and in so doing, renders the sufferers anywhere on the scale of uncomfortable (this might show itself with a flare up of Eczema), to severely ill and in extreme cases it can cause an Anaphylactic Reaction, which, if not treated appropriately, may cause death!!!

Eczema and Allergies can leave the sufferer and the parents or carers feeling helpless, frustrated, stressed and often scared.

This book will walk you through some of the treatments we tried and the effects they had on my son – both good and bad. The diary extracts are from the first seven months of my son's life when I faced a new fight trying to understand and eventually battle these overwhelming and stressful conditions.

Finally, I couldn't imagine that my son and I had suffered like this for so long, just for the experience of it, so we had to put it in writing and give it out to the world.

Foreword

by
Marie-Ange Martincic

Jayden and his mother Fredericka came to Spa Centre (The Cure) one morning in September 2003 ... I remember well their entry into the hall of the Baths ... this little angel and his mom, shy, sublime, both moving in this curious mixture of anxiety, inquisitiveness and hope.

Like many families of children with atopic Eczema at the Spa Centre, their suffering is palpable. So many difficult nights and so many daily stresses where every day is a fight with or against the skin. All this can be read on their faces.

The smile we give is the first step which is reassuring. It is essential for the team of staff and Health practitioners at the Spa Centre to be respectful, understanding and tolerant. It is through this that we look to maintain a harmony between all the skin diseases that will be presented to us. The Cure is a time to talk, listen, meet and understand without judging.

In this atmosphere, the Centre has hosted many other forms of support to thousands of families over the years whilst providing assistance and education in all areas. Practical advice and information are structured in the form of workshops and conferences, to deliver important messages to help sufferers and carers learn how to handle this daily and constant experience with Eczema and other skin disease.

At the Spa we must be modest, it's the Water, Avène Thermal Spring Water from the depths of the Earth, which gives us the healing through its soothing and anti-irritant qualities, the smiles and the joy found as a renaissance for these children and families is because of the water. The guestbook at the entrance to the Spa is full of messages each year so emotionally charged that they invite us to understand our human condition and be more modest.

It is the experience from the Spa that brings hope and massive benefits. We must thank Fredericka and Jayden for sharing theirs. They are the ones whose lives have been enriched. We are grateful that we can be a part of making the very difficult and stressful lives of the sufferers and their carers more comfortable and hopeful. This book tells a typical story.

Director, Avène Spa, France

Disclaimer

The purpose of this book is to promote awareness, education and communication on the vast range of choices, decisions and stresses regarding Eczema and Allergies. This book is not intended to replace the services of trained Health Professionals, neither is it intended to be a substitute for the medical advice of a Doctor, GP, Dermatologist or other experts. The medications and forms of treatments mentioned in this book are stated to take you on our journey as we battled with Eczema and Allergies.

Furthermore, any product or remedy discussed does not imply special endorsement or recommendation.

Medical advice should be sought before any changes in Eczema or Allergy treatments are made.

All information was correct at the time of publishing.

Introduction

My baby son Jayden was clinically diagnosed with Eczema by the time he was two months old. Before then, his condition was called 'dry skin'. My baby was uncomfortable, irritatable, sore and very unhappy. By the age of one his Eczema was diagnosed as 'severe!'

In addition to Eczema, I suspected he had Allergies and many food intolerances, but I had no 'clinical proof' of this. For almost two years I struggled to convince the doctors that something else was wrong. By December 2002 when he was almost 2 years old it was official, he did in fact have multiple Allergies! As well as this, I had noted a number of food intolerances, but because they were not proven through clinical tests, I was looked at suspiciously and there are letters to my GP from a Consultant highlighting, "...the list of intolerances are extensive and entirely from his mother...'. I guessed he was saying my suspicions were unfounded...

I had always seen myself as a solution finder, but this time I couldn't do it, I couldn't fix things for my baby. I felt so helpless because I, his mother, was supposed to be able to make everything better, but I just didn't know how to.

My story begins with a desperate search for answers to questions that no one seemed to be able to give me:

> How do I help my baby?
> How do I stop his itching?
> Why do certain foods affect him so badly?
> Why did this happen?
> Is sleep too much to ask for?

This book tells the story of our battle with Eczema and Allergies. My hope is that in doing so, it will highlight the struggles that millions of parents/carers are going through every day. I write as a mother and not as a Medical Professional or a qualified Health Practitioner. I have been with my son every step of the way – what is written on each of these pages is what we have been through, with extracts from my personal diaries.

By coming on this journey with us you will see the predicaments we faced, some of them desperate, the solutions we came up with and where we are today. If you are facing your own battles with Eczema and Allergies right now, in your child's life, my hope is that you will be able to draw parallels, be comforted, encouraged, strengthened and gain knowledge by reading our story.

> There is hope and there are alternatives.
> You are not alone.

I have become quite excellent in my Health and Fitness role and in the 1990's my expert skills landed me many lucrative opportunities and this enabled me to purchase my first house whilst I was studying for my Degree. Ten years into the industry and I had a very comfortable and happy life.

One of my dreams was to settle down and have children - I got married and after one year the plan was to get pregnant, work as long as I could up to the birth, then take 6 months off with baby. Well that was my plan... The planned 6 months became almost 4 years away from full time work!!!

My background in Health and Fitness together with patience and hope were needed when my baby was born. My pregnancy was a good one with just a couple of scares. The first came at week 10 when I began bleeding. Investigations quickly showed that there was not anything wrong. Some women bleed during pregnancy and go on to have successful pregnancies, and thank God I was one of them. The bleeding was resolved by week 15.

At week 26 the second scare had me admitted to hospital for 3 days observation. I suffered from Fibroids and they were growing as my baby grew, this caused me to have pain and contractions. After things calmed down I was discharged with a prescription to of Co-

Dydramol (a strong pain killer) to take for the rest of my pregnancy. I took the prescription for one day only after I got home because the medication was affecting my baby and making him very still. Fortunately, the pain went and the rest of the pregnancy was pain-free and fun.

Physically, there were no more problems, however my mother-in-law, Christine Denis was very ill with cancer. She was a very special lady who did the best she could with all she had. I loved her very much. She died in November 2000 leaving a gap in my life. This was a sad time, my child would never meet either of his amazing Grandmothers.

Despite these setbacks, I loved being pregnant, I found it fascinating and a blessing. I was excited about seeing my baby but a little anxious about giving birth, however I didn't concentrate on that part. My focus was on enjoying all the moments of him growing inside of me.

Having my baby

February 20th was my due date and that date came and went without event. On February 22nd I was called to hospital where the Consultant broke my waters and sent me home. I felt so excited, at last this present wrapped up inside of me for months was going to be revealed.

I was told to expect to go into labour that evening ..... I didn't.

Friday, February 23rd at around 10pm contractions start but they are in my lower spine. It's not where I expected them to be, I expected them to be in my stomach. The contractions come every few minutes and they feel as if they are trying to separate my spine both outwards and upwards, the intensity takes my breath away... I cannot think, speak or breathe whilst in the grip of a contraction. When it ceases, it leaves no trace that it was ever there, wow!! That is what you call pain!

I go to the hospital and I am put on a monitor. I am told I have a long way to go, as I am only dilated a couple of centimetres and I should go home and return when the pain gets really intense. I say that the pain *is* already intense. A Midwife with zero people skills tells me 'if you think this is pain you should wait until your labour really kicks in, then you will really know about it'. WHAT!!! She has filled me with fear and I cannot imagine the pain being much worse than it is now. I surrender to the fact that this is going to be an ordeal and all my meditation and positive thoughts throughout the pregnancy have left with her flippant comment, but I also know there is no turning back. I comfort myself with the knowledge that millions of women give birth every day, my mother did it seven times! I could definitely do it once.

I go home and sit in a bath filled with warm water and Lavender, it's a beautiful contrast to the cold February night. When the bath can no longer relieve my pain, I walk up and down, finally exhausted I rock myself on my bed trying to sleep – I cannot.

Early the next morning at around 5am I am out of bed, I walk up and down in my bathroom. When the contractions begin, I hold onto the frame of the window staring out of it, looking at the birds flying from branch to branch with no thought of what I'm going through. I imagine that life for them is just normal, they don't know I'm here. My pain is just too bad and when it comes I can hardly breathe, so all the breathing exercises I've learned about in prenatal classes fly out of the window to join the birds on the branches.

I return to the hospital that morning, Saturday February 24th, I am partly dilated so I'm admitted. I say I want an Epidural even though my Birth Plan was to 'give birth with gas and air and the deep controlled breathing I was taught'. No way! I need an Epidural now! The Anaesthetist is called and I have to wait for ages because he is busy with another mother-to-be.

My labour is horrendous. I did not imagine that pain could be so strong. I feel I might easily die right there on the bed. The contractions come and go and I am still not fully dilated, I'm waiting for that to happen. Eventually I am given a drug to help the process. When the contractions come my baby's heart rate keeps lowering. The midwives and doctors are concerned about why this is happening. They use a scalpel like instrument and keep scraping the top of my baby's head to get blood to check he is getting enough oxygen - he is. I feel concerned because the scalpel has my baby's hair on it as well as blood. 'You must be hurting him', I say. They tell me they need the readings and my baby is fine. Why would they say that? They are cutting his head!

The Anaesthetist arrives and I have to sit very still for him to put a long needle into my spine, this is difficult because the time between contractions are getting shorter. When a break in my contractions comes he does the job quickly. I didn't plan on having an Epidural, I wanted to have my baby as naturally as possible. That doesn't matter now, I just want to have my baby. After the Epidural is in place, I can breathe, why hadn't I done this all along? I cannot feel any pain, just a tightening feeling from the contractions, what a relief. The problem now is for the next 20 or so hours I struggle to give birth, it's difficult to push because I cannot really feel much below my waist. The Epidural is topped up whenever I say I feel a little pain.

At around 2.30am the following day, 25th February it is decided that I need to be taken to the Theatre. I ask why and they say they need to prepare me for a Caesarean because the baby cannot get around my cervix and I have been in labour for too long. I ask 'is my baby in danger' they say no. I ask 'am I in danger', they say no. I insist I do not want a Caesarean. They say I should go to the Theatre just in case. I start to cry, I can't believe it, you mean to say that after all this work I have to have a Caesarean? No way! I ask if I can stay where I am for a while longer and they agree I can. What do I have to do? They tell me I need to push but I cannot feel to push. I imagine I am doing the last rep of a very difficult set of squats in the gym and my baby moves further down, this is progress. Next I am cut, then a Ventouse is used, it looks like a plunger and it sucks onto the top of my baby's tiny head (which doesn't feel so tiny at all) and pulls him out. After 24 hours of labour and an incision, HE IS BORN!!!! I have a son.

Hallelujah!

The umbilical cord is wrapped twice around my baby's neck. They quickly untangle him I look at him for a moment, his eyes are open and he frowns as if to say, 'what on Earth was that all about'? They take him to the side of the room to help him. I look over at my baby, however, I can't see him because he is surrounded by the doctors and nurses. I ask 'is my baby alright' they say 'yes, we are just clearing his lungs'. I am anxious to see him. I am stitched up and I hear my baby's cry, it's loud, the midwife, nurses and doctors part and I can see him. They bring my baby to me. He is so long, and beautiful. He pulls his knees up towards his chest and is put on mine. He is so perfect. I am fascinated that this perfectly formed baby has grown inside me. I cry and cry and say hello to him over and over again.

Thank you Lord.

MY DIARY

In The Beginning

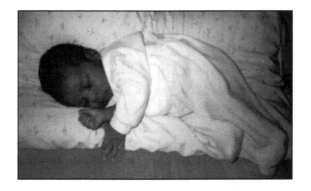

25th February 2001

24 hours of labour and my son is born – five days overdue (according to the doctors). I had to have my waters broken, be induced, have an Epidural, cut, entertained with the possibility of a Caesarean and helped with a Ventouse. It was a little traumatic... no that's not the truth, it was a VERY traumatic start to the outside world for my baby and I.

Even so, I am blessed to have had a great pregnancy and I give birth to a healthy, strong boy. He is long, alert, beautiful, and weighs eight pounds. My son is a gift from God and the start of a new chapter to my life.

He is called Baby Boy for 10 days until at last we give him the name 'Jayden' which, in Hebrew, means 'thankful', 'God has heard' and 'God will judge'.

Within two days of my baby's birth, I suspect he has Eczema because his skin is very dry with lots of rashes. The midwives assure me he is just dry from being overdue and his skin will balance itself in time.

Deep down I know it is Eczema but, they are the experts and this is my first baby so I am reassured...

Within a couple of weeks he develops Eczema and later goes on to develop internal and external intolerances and Allergies to food and other substances.

Early Signs –
Something's not quite right

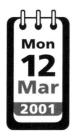

(2 weeks old)

My baby is stunning, so cute and chubby. I have been overwhelmed with well wishes and gifts. It's a very happy time and my home is constantly filled with visitors, as friends and family drop by to say hello and to see my baby. I smile and welcome them but deep down I don't want them to keep coming as I have been battling with his dry skin and sleep since birth. I'm finding it difficult to cope with the whole baby thing and every time I settle him and sit down, there is a knock on the door. I can't turn people away so I greet them and welcome them in.

Two weeks old and I haven't found anything that successfully hydrates my baby's skin without causing irritation. Olive oil helps, but not for long. After a couple of hours I notice that the oil has made his skin shiny and hot, but not moisturised.

Today he's rubbing his cheeks on whatever he can. They are cracked and look raw and a little weepy. The Health Visitor says it looks like he does have Eczema on his cheeks. "Don't worry about it", she said reassuringly, "many babies get it but it quickly clears up." I want to believe her, so I do.

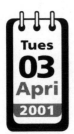 **(5 weeks old)**

Tues 03 April 2001

Five weeks since I gave birth and we haven't been able to sleep much. My baby just doesn't sleep longer than about 45 minutes. I have read that at around 4 months old most babies settle into a sleep routine and things get easier. As long as I can sleep I will be ok - I start counting down the days to 4 months.

Today he is really itchy and wiggling about. I've just fed him and he's going red. I see blotches and tiny raised spots coming up on his arms and tummy. This isn't the first time. I noticed this within a week of his birth actually, but I dismissed it as nothing major. I'm hoping it's because he is

POLLUTION AND STRESS play a big part in the condition of my son's skin. When we have travelled to Crete or Cyprus and play in the sea his condition is remarkably better. This I learned much later on.

just getting used to being out of the womb and exposed to the polluted environment of London.

Deep down I suspect he has Allergies or intolerances as well as Eczema. I don't want to think that, but I do. He is fully breastfed so I'm doing the best for him. I'm guessing that he might be reacting to what I'm eating sometimes. This doesn't make me feel good. I've got to moderate my diet so Jayden can be comfortable.

I imagined I would be a cool and relaxed mum, but I'm not. I feel like I did something wrong with my diet when I was pregnant. Maybe I had been too stressed emotionally.... Mostly my pregnancy was great, in fact, I loved it! There were just a few incidences, but everything turned out well.

Could the Co-Dydramol I had taken at 26 weeks, have adversely affected him? Maybe, I don't know. At the time I didn't think about the possible side effects, I just took what was prescribed. *During the writing of this book, I have looked at some research and the information that comes with the drug read, 'this drug is not recommended during pregnancy or breastfeeding'. Confusing...! Why give it to me?*

The third incident was at 7 months, I lost my wonderful mother-in-law. It was a devastating, very emotional and stressful time. My thoughts are, could any of these things have triggered my son's condition? Who knows! I'm looking for something to blame his condition on but in hindsight lots of members of my family have Allergies, intolerances and Eczema – not as severe as Jayden but Allergies, intolerances and Eczema nonetheless.

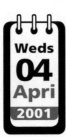 Good morning world. Perhaps I have slept for an hour. I am exhausted. My son just doesn't sleep through the night or day for that matter. On average he sleeps for around 45 minutes at a time. Maybe today will be a better one. My son has been sleeping beside me in my bed, that way I can hold his hands away from his face when he wants to rub his cheeks too much.

Weds 04 April 2001

Whilst I change his nappy I sing to him. After, I put him on my breast and he relaxes as he feeds, he is always happy and relaxed when feeding.

Often I can see the correlation between my son getting rashes and when I feed him. A few weeks back I thought the rashes might be due to the washing powder, perfume or moisturiser I use. Now I don't wear perfume, I wash our clothes in Eco Sensitive and rinse many times to ensure all the residue has gone, plus I use a hypoallergenic moisturiser on my own skin.

I've done a little research and found that babies with Eczema can be sensitive to wheat and a list of other common allergens including citrus fruit and nuts. I've always loved bread and I eat a lot of it, plus I have 'Fruit and Fibre' or 'Shreddies' cereals most mornings and drink lots of grapefruit juice. To help him I've decided to stop consuming these things thereby avoiding wheat, nuts and citrus fruit. I'll avoid them for a few days to see what happens. Maybe his rash will clear up completely. I'm hopeful.

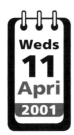

(6 weeks old)

Weds 11 Apri 2001

It might be my imagination but it's been a few days since I've decided to completely avoid wheat, nutty cereal and citrus fruit, Jayden is more comfortable, maybe a little less irritated and so am I, this is great. His skin is still very dry and he's still itchy but he looks a little better. There are still things going on with Jayden that I haven't discovered and I need to, then all will be fine. I feel like I'm getting somewhere.

I visit my doctor today and tell him that I'm excluding certain foods to help my baby and it looks like it's helping but I believe there are other things affecting him. He tells me there is no need to exclude anything because it's not possible for me to know what my baby is reacting to and I wouldn't be able to tell, not through my breast milk. I explain to him what has been happening when I eat those foods – Jayden's redness and irritability etc. My GP tells me it's probably not that, his answer makes me feel I can't possibly know. Is it just my imagination? My baby is still so young and he's adjusting to a new environment. My GP might be right but I think what I'm doing is helping him, I have to do something. I can't just watch my son struggling. I leave my GP ready to do some more research.

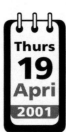 **(7 weeks old)**

Thurs 19 April 2001

I've just finished breastfeeding my son – oh my God! What's happening? His whole body is swelling up! He has hives (page 193) on his chest, tummy, back and arms and his face is a little swollen. Did I touch something and contaminate him? Oh God help me! What have I done? I am in a panic and turning around in a circle.

I dial 999 and explain what's happening. "His whole body is swollen and red. I was just feeding him..." The ambulance arrives quickly, the Paramedics give him medicine and take us to the hospital.

When we arrive at the hospital Jayden is assessed, he is now calming down, just very tired. I learn that the paramedics had given him an Antihistamine. I explain to the doctor that I thought my baby was having a reaction to the Trout I had eaten a couple of hours earlier. I'm not sure if the reaction came directly from my milk. "Well it probably didn't," he says, "It wouldn't have had time to get into your bloodstream. Maybe you touched him with something on your hand." There is no conclusion – "he could be reacting to anything".

It is the first time I have eaten Trout since Jayden was born, so I conclude it must be the Trout. I have a gut feeling. They say this is highly unlikely. I explain that often after I've fed him, he reacts by going red with those tiny raised spots; other times he would be fine. I suggest he's intolerant to some things and allergic to others. I believe he is reacting to what I eat through my milk so clearly what I am eating directly affects him. Again they imply this is highly unlikely and it's unlikely that the trout has given Jayden an allergic reaction. All I know is that I need to make him better.

Four hours later my son is discharged. Everything is back to normal, he is very sleepy.

The truth is I don't want to be right about the allergic reaction so I call this incident 'a one-off'. Even though the doctors told me not to worry about what I am eating and just continue to eat as normal, I continue to avoid wheat, nutty cereal, soya, citrus fruit and now Trout – I know he is reacting. Any one of these could be causing my son's problems. My thinking is, if only I can pinpoint the allergens and avoid them he would be cured.

To take him off my breast milk would mean that I would have to put him on some artificial formula milk and I don't think that will be the best thing for him. I have looked at the ingredients of them all and conclude that he is best off with my milk. The most commonly used infant formulas contain purified cow's milk and whey, I have a feeling, a deep down gut feeling that he will

> In 2003, the WHO and UNICEF published their Global Strategy for Infant and Young Child Feeding, it warned that "lack of breastfeeding—and especially lack of exclusive breastfeeding during the first half-year of life—are important risk factors for infant and childhood morbidity and mortality".

have a terrible reaction to milk. I am intolerant to dairy products so I will not be giving it to him. I believe he's reacting to some of the things I eat he's not reacting to my breast milk as such, he is thriving on it. I'll adjust what I eat so he can be as well and as comfortable as possible.

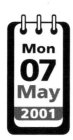

(10 weeks old)

Just over two weeks have passed since the incident with the Trout and I've got a longer list of foods that I believe my son is intolerant to. I am excluding from my diet (and therefore his, as I'm still breastfeeding): Trout, soya, wheat, citrus fruit, refined sugar, salt and hydrogenated fats.

Externally, I am only using olive oil and perfume-free moisturisers on my skin as I find that my son's skin does not react favourably to anything with perfume in it. I believe I'm doing the right thing, he is more comfortable but the problem is not resolved. He is still dry, itchy and sore. The moisturisers are not moisturising his skin. But I believe he would be worst if I didn't do the things I do.

I have again told my doctor what I have discovered concerning my baby's condition but he rejects my findings saying I have no way of knowing what he is allergic or intolerant to because my son has not had any clinical investigations. Does that make my finding worthless? He's dismissive of the fact that I have conducted my own investigations by simply being with my baby all day and all night and seeing him react. I've decided that I am not going to listen to the doctor concerning this. I am with my baby 24/7 so doesn't that make me the best person to make a judgement on this? I need to help my baby and

I need the doctors to help me do that. I feel so helpless but I need to keep on doing something to try to make things better.

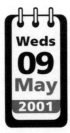

I'm at the GP yet again requesting for my son to have testing for Allergies, this is not granted. My Doc-

> "Knowing what you're allergic to is key to managing your condition," says Allergy UK's Lindsey McManus. (2004)

tor thinks that it's not necessary for my baby to have a test. He says I need to relax, my baby is so young, I need to be calm and give him time to settle. I leave the surgery understanding what my GP has asked me to do but not knowing how to do what he has asked. I feel helpless.

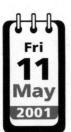

We have been up most of the night. Jayden's been scratching and crying, he is not happy and nothing I do is helping him.

By the evening I call the 'GP After Hours Surgery', a Doctor visits us at 00.30am. He writes a note to the hospital, '... Jayden is inflamed everywhere except for his thighs, flexes and bottom. He's distressed but eating well'. He is admitted to the hospital with a skin infection and given 'Augmetin', an Antibiotic. I am told to continue with his moisturisers, additionally we're pre-scribed Hydrocortisone.

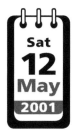

Sat 12 May 2001

My son is discharged with Hydrocortisone and Antibiotics to take for the next 5 days. In actual fact we were only at the hospital for a few hours. I'm feeling like I really need to understand what's happening with my baby but I'm not getting the answers I need to help me to help myself - I don't even know what to ask!!!

Jayden is uncomfortable for the rest of the day and all night with moments of calmness, so I am on edge all the time. When he is still, I creep around the house trying to get things done: I shower, eat, wash clothes, do research, research and more research. I feel hopeful when I'm searching to find solutions.

Over the next few days the infection seems to have cleared up. To be honest when I was told he had an infec-tion, it was a surprise. I sigh because I don't know what to do, things just keep surprising me. I'm not coping.

It's been 10 weeks since he was born and I haven't had a good night's sleep... things are feeling difficult, I'm so tired. My sister left me a message today asking if I'm alright and offering her help so I can go out or just have a rest. I send her a reply saying that I am absolutely fine. Some of my family are going out next week and she wants me to come, I will make my excuses.

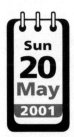 **(12 weeks old)**

I have a feeling that tomatoes are adding to my son's problems. I do enjoy them but I've read that they can cause problems in terms of allergic reactions. I have added tomatoes to my elimination list. I'll see what happens.

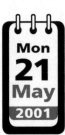 I'm back at our GP because Jayden is so restless and his skin is weepy. The GP says he is still infected. Jayden's given another course of Antibiotics. We go home and during the evening Jayden is not well. His skin is inflamed and even weepier, especially around his neck. He now has diarrhoea and a temperature so I call NHS Direct and they advise that I call an ambulance, I do... my baby is admitted to hospital. He is prescribed 48 hours of Intravenous Antibiotics and a 10 day course of Oral Antibiotics. I have three different creams that I have to apply to his skin – 50/50 paraffin in White Soft Paraffin, to help keep moisture in his skin; Hydrocortisone 0.5%, to help reduce inflammation and Nystatin Cream to help eliminate the infection.

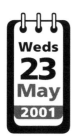

We are discharged from the hospital with the remaining course of Antibiotics and the skin creams. I go home wondering how I can ensure this doesn't happen again. What can I change? What should I add to his routine to help him? At the hospital they've told me I'm doing an excellent job and my baby is just unfortunate to have such severe Eczema.

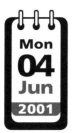

(14 weeks old)

Slept for a total of 2 hours last night. I get out of bed, change Jayden's nappy and get him dressed into some fresh clothes. He's in the kitchen with me sitting in his bouncing chair. I am standing up eating a bowl of Muesli and chatting to him. I bend down towards him and kiss him on his mouth. Within seconds his mouth is massively swollen – if it swells anymore it will burst! I flap around the room looking for the phone to call for an ambulance. But I cannot dial, I have to keep moving. I need to go to the hospital now. Oh God, help!

I said I was not going to eat anything with nuts, but here I am eating a bowl of Muesli and to add to it I've kissed him on his mouth! Have I lost my mind?! How stupid can I be?!!!

We drive frantically to the hospital pressing on the car horn constantly with the lights flashing. We don't stop at any traffic lights. We can't get to the hospital quick enough. The journey seems to take a life time but it was about 15 minutes. We rush straight up to the Children's Ward where he

> Anaphylactic shock is a serious allergic reaction that is rapid in onset and may cause death. It can result in a number of symptoms including throat swelling, an itchy rash, and low blood pressure.

was almost 2 weeks ago. The doctor tells me off and says I should have called an ambulance as Jayden could have gone into anaphylactic shock! It is suspected that he has a nut allergy.

To my knowledge we don't have any history of severe food allergies in our family. I am eager to ask my family questions to find out where this came from. My father has told me that as a child I had mild Eczema on my ankles and elbows and one of my older sisters had some major 'skin problems' as a baby. Her condition was never given an official name. She was born in Dominica in the Caribbean and my mum used to bathe her in the river there to help heal her. My mother died 18 years before I had my son so I couldn't get advice from her. I developed an intolerance to dairy products in my late twenties and some of my nieces have various food intolerances. My son's father has mild Hay Fever... so I guess we do have a history of Allergies after all, but not anything as severe as Jayden's though! Where had this come from? Why so severe? How could I have prevented this? How can I stop it? I believe that if I research deep enough I will find the answers to all these questions and then find the cure for my son. I feel optimistic.

Jayden is given 10mls of Antihistamine and the swelling quickly goes down. My baby has to stay in overnight for observation. I feel so stupid and irresponsible, I should have been more careful. NUTS FOR GOODNESS SAKE!!!

It is around 9pm and the ward is quiet and there are other parents staying with their children. I am sitting on a chair with my legs up on the bed, breastfeeding my baby, he is so sleepy. I find myself staring at the other parents, they look as if they're coping. I feel like I am fighting a war alone, having to learn all the rules from scratch by trial and error and my little baby is suffering as a result. I cry and pray, "Dear Lord, help me to be a great mum." I vow to do better. "I will do better", I whisper in my son's ear and kiss his sleepy face.

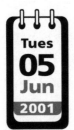

Tues 05 Jun 2001 This is the day after the storm of the nut reaction and all is calm, my baby is on my lap and I am pressing the button on his Winnie the Pooh book for the 100th time it seems, the recording says, "Oh stuff and fluff", Jayden chuckles every time, he loves this book. I use it as a distraction when he's fretful and also just to make him smile. Despite all he goes through, he smiles so much.

It is 4pm the Doctor comes around and my baby is discharged and prescribed an Antihistamine. My beautiful little bundle is released back to me to be taken home. I am determined to make a better job of this and not make a mistake like this EVER again.

I ask for an Epipen to take home – because of the major reaction he just had, I'm surprised that they didn't pack us off with one in the first instance. The Doctor says I need to speak to my GP if I think I need one. I ask 'why?' he says they have no idea what my son is reacting to and Antihistamine was all that was needed to make him better, he doesn't need an Epipen...

> Epipen is a single dose of Epinephrine, Adrenaline that you can administer to counteract a severe allergic reaction until help arrives. The Adrenaline tries to counteract the body's hypersensitive reaction to an allergen.

I understand the severity of my son's reaction and I need to carry this Epipen around with me now to potentially save his live. I express my fear, "...anything could happen between now and getting an Epipen from our GP." They say they cannot give it to me. They say that without Allergy Testing they cannot be sure that he is allergic to nuts. I tell them that I've asked our GP for the Allergy Testing and I've been refused. Still they say I need to speak to our GP. I really do not understand. What do they mean? They saw how swollen my son was when he came to the hospital the day before! He is allergic to something! I am no longer really listening because I know they are just saying 'NO'. I see this decision as incompetent. I JUST WANT AN EPIPEN AND I WANT ALLERGY TESTING!!!

Armed with the prescribed Antihistamine I leave with my son, but I am not happy. I think they are being negligent. I do not say this to them, but I am shocked at their decision. I promise my son that I will be the best I can be and it will always be good enough.

I do not want any more surprises like this. I do not want to put my son's life at risk because I did not try hard enough to do the right thing. I could not bear that. But I don't know what the right thing is... Help me Lord... I question myself. Was I overreacting? Was this a one off, out of the blue thing that will never happen again?

I hope so. I pray so. Deep down I know it's not a one off, he had a severe reaction with Trout a few weeks before. It is from this point that I really begin pushing for Jayden to be tested for allergies.

(16 weeks old)

Mon 18 Jun 2001 Our GP will not prescribe an Epipen. Neither will he agree to Allergy Testing. I have described what happened when he came into contact with nuts and he has the report from the hospital but still he will not let me have one. He says they cannot be sure the reaction was from nuts but, I'm sure it was!!! What more do they want?!!! Why not prescribe it anyway - better safe than sorry...!!!

Allergy Testing is important as it can measure the level of allergic reaction to a variety of substances. With this information, an Action Plan can be devised so that the patient doesn't come into contact with the offending allergen, thereby avoiding the trauma experienced.

It wasn't until Jayden was almost two years old that he was tested for allergies. I don't understand why it took so long. Previously doctors were not convinced Jayden had allergies, they thought I was an over-reactive mum! At his first testing they found he was allergic to tomatoes, kiwi, lemon, salmon and trout, just as I had said. It was at this point that the Epipen was prescribed. I'm glad I stuck to my convictions.

Of course I avoid nuts – they are now not allowed in my home – but what if he comes into contact with them accidentally? I feel anxious and

paranoid when people come to visit. I do not want anyone to touch him. It seems that all of a sudden everyone
who sees him wants to touch his cheeks or kiss him.
Hasn't anyone been listening to me? Can't they see his
face is sore? Can't they see his cheeks are weeping, red
and angry?

"Please don't touch his face" I say. 'Please don't touch
him at all', is what I want to say, but I don't. You see I'm
afraid they will make him worse. Not everyone is happy
about my requests – some roll their eyes, others sympa-
thise, but I really do not care. I need to protect my son.
I have talked about his Allergies to all those around him
but some really don't realise the severity of his condition
– they think I am an 'over-cautious mum' who isn't coping very well with her first child. Well no one says that to
me... I think they think that.

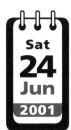

Sat
24
Jun
2001

(17 weeks old)

My baby's cheeks
are weepy so I am
using breast milk
to cleanse them.
I have been trying lots of
different moisturisers too
because when I find something
that works well, it is a matter of weeks, sometimes days,

Breast milk is excellent
and calming, it has immu-
nologic agents and other
compounds that take
action against viruses and
parasites. Breast milk is
sterile, anti-bacterial and
can help heal wounds –
it can even help people
heal faster after organ
transplants and
other surgeries!
www.Breastfeeding-
problems.com

before it becomes irritating to him, then I need to find something else.

Jayden slept 3 hours in total today, my baby's exhausted and so am I.

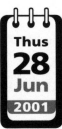
Thus
28
Jun
2001

I've been getting pressure from the Health Centre and my GP to wean Jayden off my breast milk. Can't they just leave me alone? I know my son's benefiting from my breast milk and if I start weaning him now, when I can't be sure what he's intolerant or allergic to, things are going to be even worse for him. I want more time – he needs more time before he consumes other foods. He needs time for his digestive system to develop, this I had read somewhere during my research.

My research shows that in some countries mothers are encouraged to breastfeed for the first two years, so I'm con-

"The important thing is to do what feels right for you and your baby. Continuing to breastfeed helps to reduce the chance of food intolerances and continues to protect your baby from infections, regardless of whether he is four months or two years old. The World Health Organisation recommends breastfeeding for up to two years and beyond. The longer you breastfeed, the longer the good health effects will be for you and your child".

vinced it is perfectly fine, acceptable and healthy for me to continue at this time.

I cannot begin to imagine the effect weaning will have on my baby if I do this now. He is only four months old... he has time. Why are these people hassling me?

The Health Centre thinks differently they say he's a little underweight and if I wean him now he will put on weight and meet all the centile goal posts stated in 'The Red Book'. I feel pressurised from these 'experts' on my doorstep so I take their advice and begin weaning my baby. Everything I've tried is making him vomit. I did feel this would be too early! However, they are the experts and they are right in my face but I need to be stronger and more confident with my decisions. I am following all the recommendations for weaning, still Jayden is managing to keep down only about 10 percent of it. I am not feeling really worried about him getting enough other foods because he is thriving on my milk. However, I'm not happy he's vomiting so often. Apart

> THE RED BOOK is the Personal Child Health Record book you are given at the Health Centre when you have a baby. This book contain sections to record whether or not your child is reaching all the 'goal posts' set by the authorities, i.e. weight, height, alertness and so on. There is also a page with all the recommended immunisations and at what stage your child should have them.

from the Allergies and Eczema my baby is healthy and alert so what's the big deal? To reassure myself I contact breastfeeding institutions who say it would be fine and beneficial to purely breastfeed him for the first year, especially as he has Eczema and Allergies.

I am confident he is getting his nutrients. Today I have decided I will take my time and wean him slowly. I try not to feel hassled or pressurised by the 'experts' however, I do. It's obvious to me that my baby has other intolerances and Allergies that I have not identified yet.

Skin Infection and Steroids

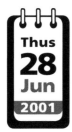

Thus 28 Jun 2001

This week we have visited our GP every day. I am sitting in the waiting room with my baby as his skin is shedding before my eyes! Whenever he moves his head his skin brushes off onto my clothes, it's a mess. I don't want anyone to look at him. I think it's because, I don't want them to think I'm not taking care of him well enough. I'm not sure. I feel very conscious of the fact that his skin is so sore, dry and flaky and I can't fix it. I feel guilty about that, I think. I'm having to moisturise him about every 20 minutes! His skin just doesn't seem to keep moisturise in. Presently I'm getting through about 500g of moisturiser a week.

Often his skin sheds so completely that underneath would be fresh and clear, in my ignorance and optimism I hope he has shed all the Eczema and he'd be ok. But, no he isn't ok! The fresh skin would scale up again and the process would begin all over again.

I'm desperate for solutions and I feel the health system is failing us, and so I believe it's all up to me. In my distress I feel that not even God can help me, I've prayed but He hasn't fixed this. I have to make it alright because this must be all my fault. I don't understand why and I want to know why – there must be a why! One day, hopefully, I will know the answer. Our GP prescribes more Steroids and we go home.

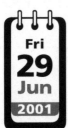

Fri
29
Jun
2001

Today we are at the GP yet again. I suspect my baby has another skin infection because his odour is different and the backs of his little knees are bleeding and weeping very slightly. Before I even take a seat or say a word, my GP looks at me and sighs as if to say, 'What is it now, woman?' (This was probably the insecurities I had developed but I felt I was a burden because I couldn't sort this out myself). Being at the GP so often makes me feel helpless but I don't know what else to do. I want to lay on the floor flat out on my face and cry 'help me!' but I can't lose control. I've got to cope, at least on the outside, inside, I am not doing so well.

> **SPECIALIST HELP**
> Looking back I can see how desperate I was. I can now sympathise with our GP. He was probably as frustrated as me. He really wasn't able to help me in the way I needed. I wanted the Eczema to be gone. I was told by a Consultant that in all the training a GP gets, only a very short time is dedicated to Dermatology. I believe it's a good idea for GP's to refer patients, to other Specialists early on.

He examines my son, agrees with me that Jayden has another infection and prescribes a five-day course of Antibiotics. We go home. I feel guilty that his skin is infected again. I clean my hands well enough, don't I? Sorry my baby. Jayden doesn't sleep well but this is not unusual. He wriggles, scratches and cries a lot and when at last he falls asleep, I can't sleep because he's scratching in his sleep. I put cotton mittens on his hands to protect him from his scratching however, he gets them off. I stitch the mittens to his sleeves. He rubs whatever he can. He is so uncomfortable and hot and he will do whatever he needs to do to relieve his discomfort.

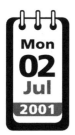

(18 weeks)

Mon 02 Jul 2001

I'm sitting in the GP surgery again. I am worried about the extreme shedding of my son's skin. The Doctor tells me this is what Eczema does and I should continue with the moisturisers, bath additives and emollients previously prescribed. I tell him about the reservations I have concerning the Steroids. I think they will damage my baby's skin. He reassures me that they will help by reducing inflammation in the long term.

> Topical Steroids are applied to the skin in the form of creams, ointments and lotions and prescribed to control flare-ups of Eczema and other inflamed skin conditions.

I am reluctant to use the Steroids as I find it makes my son's skin even redder and inflamed almost the moment I put it on him. My conclusion is 'it does not agree with him'. Reluctantly, I use it because I am assured it is not hurting him. I probably need to give it more time to make a difference, only then will I really know.

He has a particularly itchy day and night time is horrendous. Tonight he is so unhappy, he's tired, fed up and he can't stop scratching. I put on a video of 'Winnie the Pooh', this always helps him. We have quite a large collection of 'Winnie the Pooh' videos now.

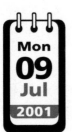

(19 weeks)

Mon
09
Jul
2001

We are back at the GP Surgery. My baby's skin has not improved, the infection is still there. The Doctor tells me this is common with Eczema and prescribes yet another course of Antibiotics! I do not want to give it to him. I believe too many Antibiotics are harmful to the body, but what choice do I have? Do I have an alternative? The doctor says I do not. He stresses the importance of my son using the Antibiotics otherwise he could get blood poisoning. Of course I need to give it to him.

I take the prescription to the chemist and my son begins yet another five-day course of Antibiotics. He scratches for most of the day and sleeps only 45-minute stretches tonight - as usual. We are exhausted.

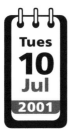 I am back at the GP surgery telling him that I've stopped using the Steroids prescribed a few weeks ago as I'm concerned it makes my son's skin inflamed, red and sore. I think he is intolerant to it, so I only used it for a couple of days. He says that I would not be able to tell if he was intolerant to it after only a few applications and I should give it a few more days. I tell him I could tell he was not happy with it immediately I put it on. The Doctor is not listening to me, I am not listening to him since he's not interested in hearing what I have got to say. So much of Jayden's skin is cracked, sore, peeling and open – it can't be healthy having the Steroids going straight

Long-term side effects of Steroids Doctors often say, "We don't know the cause of Eczema, no one does", yet Steroids are widely used in the treatment to 'speed up healing'. Some Naturopathic Practitioners say Steroids suppress the disease and push it back into the body causing it to affect internal organs and create other problems.

I'm no expert in this field but this information caused me to think about the effects of drugs on the user. Were the medicines being given to heal or just to calm and mask the symptoms for the moment? I believe the latter. I was not convinced that Steroids were any good for my son.

into his bloodstream like that. I don't want to use the Steroids, I won't use it.

(19 weeks)

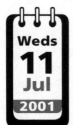

Weds 11 Jul 2001

My baby isn't well. Since our visit to the GP yesterday he's been quiet and tired. He has a temperature and his skin looks sore all over. 'Oh my little baby, what can I do to help you?' It looks like he's sweating all over. His body is glistening and sticky. He is just lying in his nappy because he is hot. He isn't scratching today, he seems too exhausted and weak to move. I am worried and I'm lying with him, I will not take my eyes off him. I don't think he's alright at all. I go to pick him up but he's stuck to the sheet so I slowly peel him off. His skin is weeping all over. It seems to be seeping – even on his back where he doesn't have Eczema!

I later learn that long-term Steroid use can cause skin thinning and a list of other side effects. I have a friend who suffered with Eczema for most of her childhood. She is now 70 years old and has major skin problems on her hands because of extensive use of Steroids which have made her skin very thin so it cuts and tears easily.

She advised me to be very careful with it. It's true that I didn't know how often she used it but it was enough for me to know that I didn't want to put my son at risk.

I call the GP – it's late, so I'm put through to an emergency number. I explain what has been happening in a panicked state. A Doctor quickly arrives at our home. He assesses my baby and says he needs to be admitted to hospital as an emergency. He has lost a lot of fluid and his skin is infected. I explain what's happened over the last week and that he started another course of Antibiotics two days ago. I feel I need to let him know I'm a good mother. I didn't neglect my son. He says not to worry and that this is common for babies with severe Eczema. He proceeds to call an ambulance to take us to the local hospital.

Specialist Hospital

In the process of my research I've learnt that Guys and St Thomas's Hospital in London have a Specialist Dermatology Department for Children. It has a reputation of excellence. I ask the Doctor if we can be taken there instead. He says the ambulance will only take us to our local hospital but he will gladly give us a letter for the hospital of our choice, however, we would have to make our own way there - so we do. I wrap my son up in a sheet, I call a taxi, quickly pack a bag and we are off.

Upon arrival at Guys and St Thomas's Hospital we are seen almost immediately. My son is wrapped in his sheet with only his nappy on. The sheet is slowly peeled off him to reveal his sore and weepy skin.

My son is weak and sleepy. The nurse looks at me. She is asking me some questions. Then she asks, "Can I have the name of his Social Worker please?" I start looking through my son's papers and I pull out a sheet with the information I think the nurse is requesting.

"No, not his Health Visitor," she says.
"Does he have a Social Worker?" I now understand.
"Why would my son have a Social Worker?",
I say defensively.
"He has a skin infection, he has severe Eczema;
what are you talking about?!"

I'm imagining she thinks I've neglected my baby. Deep down I believe I have done something wrong for my baby to be in this condition. I am being careful and doing the best I can. I don't feel happy about this question. I ask her again why my baby would need a Social Worker. She says it's just a routine question. She smiles, I leave it. I want to cry and shout out that I am doing my best but I can't get on top of this and I need them to help me to sort this out once and for all! I need different help but I feel insecure about the fact that I feel I'm not coping. I hold in my frustrations and desperation and get on with the job of communicating calmly.

Treatment

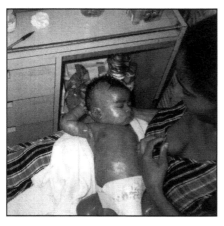

Jayden is seen by a Doctor who tells me that he will need to be admitted. His treatment is an intravenous drip of Antibiotics and 50/50 Emollient. We are at the mercy of the Doctors once again. I believe they will help him and he'll be fine.

Numbing cream is applied to the back of Jayden's tiny little hand and a short while later a Cannula is inserted, he protests by wriggling and crying. The procedure is hurting him. He looks at me as if to say, 'Mummy, why are you allowing them to do this to me?' I hold him close to me while the needle is inserted. His hand is bandaged all the way up to his shoulder and there is a splint at his elbow so he cannot bend his arm and try to take the needle out. He protests some more. Now he is completely exhausted and so am I.

> A Cannula is a hollow surgical needle used to create a temporary entry to a vein or artery so that drugs can be given intravenously to a patient at any time without having to repeatedly puncture the patient's skin.

My job is to apply the 50/50 emollient to his whole body to stop moisture leaving him (I believe that's why), I'm familiar with the product. The moment the emollient evaporates, I apply more. It makes

> 50/50 Emollient is a skin preparation made up of 50% soft white paraffin and 50% liquid paraffin used to soften and moisturise dry skin.

my son's skin hot. I also have to ensure he doesn't knock the Cannula out of his hand. This is a full time job.

Hospital Stay

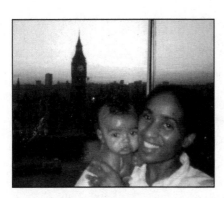

We are given an ensuite room with a single bed and a cot. The room overlooks the River Thames at Westminster and we can see Big Ben from our window. It is a beautiful, peaceful scene of London at night which is just as well because the curtain rail is broken so I can't draw it. I would pay big money to have a cosy hotel room with this beautiful view. I show Jayden the sites, I want him to know it all. I want him to have the best of the best. I will remember this, he won't, he's only a baby. I kiss him and pray that God will guide and help me to give my son the best of everything.

It's 1:00am, the Nurses and Doctors have left us and all is quiet. I sit on the bed with my son fast asleep in my arms. I stare out of the window, I'm alone again. I wonder how I could have prevented this from happening. I cry for my baby's pain and ask God for help to be able to do better. I place my baby into the cot beside my bed and lay on my bed staring at him until I drift off to sleep.

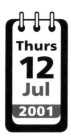 Jayden woke up three times during the night but only for a short time, thank God. I think he feels so much more comfortable, God bless my little baby, he was exhausted. The Doctors and Nurses have been brilliant.

Thurs 12 Jul 2001

8:00am and the sun is shining in through the window and the room is bright. By midday the room is hot – too hot! I wouldn't otherwise complain, I love the sun, but Eczema and heat do not agree so this is not the ideal environment. I can't shut the sun out because the curtain rail is broken. We are given a big electric fan to keep my son cool. It is rickety and loud, but it does the job.

In the early afternoon we walk around the ward where we see so many children with serious health problems. My heart goes out to them and their parents and I pray for them. I thank God for everything. I know one day

He will let us understand and all of this will be clear. I have a moment of extreme calmness, clarity and gratefulness for all we have been through.

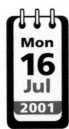 It's six days after being admitted to Guys and St Thomas's. During our time here the Doctors and Nurses have been supportive. I am still breastfeeding so there isn't any food for the hospital to prepare for Jayden. The food I am given is good. We sometimes go out and walk along the riverside, the weather and the fresh air is lovely. It's been good staying here because we are taken care of and I don't need to think about all the other things my life at home demands.

Today we are going home. The Paediatric Nurse has just taken the bandage off Jayden's arm and removed the Cannula. His arm and hand look puffy and pale and the skin feels soggy, however he's relieved it's off. He wriggles and bends his arm in celebration it seems. God bless him, he is a Champion. "You're my inspiration Jayden", I tell him.

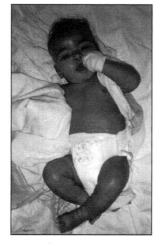

We leave the hospital with a follow-up appointment for four weeks time and go home in a cab. When we arrive at our front door I feel relieved, and I sense Jayden is too. He giggles and kicks his legs when we get into his room. He recognioses we are home and he's very happy to see all his toys and familiar surroundings, he is delighted.

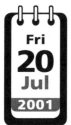

(20 weeks)

**Fri
20
Jul
2001**

It's been four days since we left the hospital. My son's neck is weeping in the creases again. I can detect that familiar odour again - the infection is back!!! Just like the Doctor predicted, but it's localised. I have been careful to wash my hands and keep Jayden clean. I can't keep on top of this! Surely I can apply something directly to his skin and zap it, but what?

I go to our GP and he confirms Jayden's skin is infected again, or maybe it didn't quite clear up from the last time. Either way he needs another course of Antibiotics. I don't want to give this to Jayden. He's just spent all that time at the hospital on Intravenous Antibiotics, that didn't fully work! I ask the GP if there is something else I can do, he says no. He tells me the importance of giving Jayden the Antibiotics again to clear this up, if I don't he could get very sick. Oh my God!!!

I'm in a dilemma, I know I have to give this to him, but if I keep giving him Antibiotics I could make his immune system vulnerable in the future. I express my concerns to the Doctor, he says I have no choice. I go back to the hospital we were just discharged from for a second opinion. They give me the same news. The Doctor goes on to explain that because of the severity of Jayden's Eczema this will happen often. I am not happy with this prediction and I quietly reject the statement. It's my mission this will not happen often, not to my son, I will find a way, it's now my project. There must be something I can do so that Jayden won't have to keep taking Antibiotics that means I need to ensure he doesn't keep getting skin infections.

I take the prescription and get the medicine from the chemist. I go home but I don't give the medicine to Jayden immediately. I give myself two hours to find a solution. If I don't find something in this time I'll give the Antibiotics to him.

He is safe for now.

Naturopathic Practitioner

I sit at the computer with the Antibiotics in front of me. I need to find an alternative, because the infection is only on his neck. If it was as serious as it was previously when he was admitted, I would give him the Antibiotics immediately, however this doesn't seem major. There must be something else I can use. After an hour of surfing remedies I decide I need to speak to someone about it. There are so many websites offering potions to cure – I have already spent hundreds of pounds online and the products do not live up to their promises. I don't want to part with my money without being as sure as possible. I need something to help my son NOW! I am desperate but feel confident that I will discover something today and I don't want the remedy to be more internal Antibiotics, not today.

I find a place online that specialises in Naturopathy, I call the number and speak to a lady called Vanessa about our situation. I make an appointment and two hours later Jayden and I arrive at her apartment in Canary Wharf, not too far from where we live. When we enter the apartment, Jayden's face lights up and he seems totally happy as he focus' on a large poster of his favourite character, 'Winnie the Pooh' hanging on the wall. There are also two large stuffed Winnie the Pooh toys in the consultation room. My baby is happy and calm in this place.

Tea Tree Oil has a long history of positive, traditional uses. Australian aboriginals use tea tree leaves for healing skin cuts, burns, and infections by crushing the leaves and applying them to the affected area.

There have been many times when Jayden's skin has been sore and cracked open, at times like these, his skin is vulnerable to infection so we use the oil everyday during this period. It's a simple remedy but please be advised that I am not recommending you use this in the place of Antibiotics which have a role to play in infection. Always seek sound medical advice.

Vanessa is a Naturopathic Practitioner. At the cost of £60 an hour she does a consultation and recommends that I put a drop of Tea Tree Oil in Jayden's bath every day. She says Jayden's skin is not severely infected and that I do not need to give the prescribed Antibiotics at this time. She advises that this treatment would help keep his skin infection free in the future and fight the infection he has right now. The infection would clear in a few days. I am happy about this.

On the way home we make a diversion and go to Apple Jacks, Health Store in Stratford and purchase a bottle of Tea Tree Essential Oil. As soon as we get home I get online and read more about Tea Tree Oil. A short while later I run a little bath and add the Tea Tree Oil, it smells pleasant and I pray that it will take the infection away. By the next morning his neck is no longer weeping. I put one drop in his bath every day after that – this was to become the solution that killed the skin infection forever - It has never returned! Coincidence? I don't think so.

Jayden became a regular cli-ent of Vanessa's and so she learns all about him, including the exclusions I have made in his diet and why. She under-stands and supports what I had done and what I am doing and gives me some ideas about 'calm foods' to feed him. She

Calm foods are foods that do not require the digestive system to work too hard. Some of the calm foods that Vanessa suggested included green vegetables, lentils, pumpkin and squash.

explains that the skin is an indication of what is going on inside the body. He needs foods that will hydrate his system. She explains that his digestive system is prob-ably not fully developed and I should only feed him calm foods and continue with the breastfeeding for as long as I feel it is necessary.

Vanessa confirmed that people react uniquely to differ-ent things and it's as simple as that. After spending time with her, I feel a great calmness, but I also have a 'freak out' moment on the idea that food can be a killer for one person or a lifesaver for another. Of course, I knew this already but I now understand it in the context of my baby

– a Trout meal can be of great nutritional value for one person but it can kill another! This revelation drives me to make an active effort to learn about foods that can help my baby's condition and boost his immune system so he will be armed with the ability to fight anything. This fuels me and gives me a sense of empowerment. I have a definite project, a purpose and this drives me.

More allergic reactions (the GP's getting fed up)

(6 months old)

Tues
02
Aug
2001

My baby is almost six months old and I've started taking him to a Parent and Babies Morning group at our local nursery. It's a lovely place, Jayden especially likes the sensory room, so we're in there. After 30 minutes we go into the main room and sit at the snack table, he's on my lap as I'm looking at the foods he might try. We are restricted to rice cakes and raisins that I supply, however there is fruit on the table and a piece of Kiwi is placed in front of all the babies. My son picks up a piece and quickly puts it down again. I didn't think anything of it. I imagine he doesn't like the way it feels. He then rubs his cheek and within seconds his face and hand are swollen, I know it's the Kiwi. I wash his hands and face, give him 5mls of Antihistamine, put him in his buggy and leave the nursery in a hurry.

> **ANTIHISTAMINE**
> In allergic reactions, special allergy cells in the body release chemicals called Histamine. Histamine causes rashes, sneezing, itching, swelling and other allergic symptoms which can become life threatening by blocking the airways. Antihistamines stop the Histamine from working in the body, thereby reversing this extreme reaction.

We get home in less than 10 minutes as I've jogged all the way. I run a cool bath and put him straight into it. I don't go to the hospital, I take care of my baby myself now as much as possible. That was a definite allergic reaction to the Kiwi fruit and I didn't need an Allergy Test to confirm that! It's funny, I didn't realise you could be allergic to Kiwi fruit! I had heard about the common allergic reactions – dairy products, eggs and nuts – but I didn't know there were others. It sounds so silly but up until now I had no reason to think about it because I'd never known anyone with severe allergic reactions to food. I know about intolerances as I am intolerant to dairy products and some of my family members have various other food intolerances to nuts, wheat, dairy and mango, but we have no major food allergy sufferers. I do some research on the internet and find that there are a growing number of people suffering from Kiwi fruit allergy – of course you can be allergic to anything at all! I add Kiwi to the 'untouchables' list.

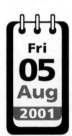 Today I feel our GP is frustrated by our frequent visits and requests for help. He looks me straight in the eyes, shakes his head and says, 'I've just had to tell a mother and father that their child has liver cancer.' I don't remember his exact words but I remember feeling sick to my stomach, sick at myself for not being able to cope. My heart went out to that child and the

family. Eczema is not a life-threatening disease, was he right? Am I being ridiculous? I leave the surgery feeling quite pathetic and vow never to return.

We still need help and expertise but it is now clear that we are not going to get what we need from our GP. I needed to do more research about how to treat my son's Allergies and Eczema.

I feel reassured when I remember meeting a Consulting Dermatologist who told me that he believed the stress suffered by parents of children with Eczema is as high as the stress suffered by parents of children with Leukaemia – wow!!! He was supportive and said that Eczema can be extremely difficult to treat in many sufferers and the lack of sleep and the helplessness felt is a problem in itself. After recalling this conversation I feel justified in all my actions. I know I am a loving mother having a normal response to my baby's desperate condition. I need to put how I feel about what my GP said in perspective, it must be difficult for him.

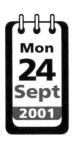

Mon
24
Sept
2001

(7 months old)

Today my baby is admitted to Homerton Hospital in East London, I've taken him there because he has been vomiting, he has diarrhoea and his nose is so blocked he's finding it difficult to breathe. Shortly after we arrive he's diagnosed with a chest infection and Rickets is also suspected, to confirm this diagnosis they give him blood tests and an X-ray. Rickets is confirmed! The blood tests

> RICKETS is a deficiency disease resulting from a lack of Vitamin D commonly due to insufficient exposure to sunlight. In children it is often characterised by defective bone growth.

also show that he is deficient in Calcium and Iron. OH MY GOD WHAT HAVE I DONE TO MY SON?

I am told off by Doctors who say I'm not feeding my son properly, that's why he has all these deficiencies. They go on to say that because he wasn't diagnosed with all the Allergies and intolerances I have listed I should feed him everything apart from nuts, "your beliefs are putting your son's health at risk!" I am confused and scared because of what's happening, I'm doing my best for my son but I'm making him ill? Oh dear God!

After just one night in the hospital my baby is discharged with a prescription of Vitamin D and I am told to go home and give him dairy products. 'Rice pudding and yogurt would be a good start', they say. They say I am depriving him of vital nutrients because of my 'strange beliefs and reasonings' concerning Jayden's condition. It is true my son has not reacted to dairy products before, because I have never given it to him, but I am sure he will react negatively if I do. There isn't any scientific reasoning for my decision, it is just a gut feeling, mother's instinct maybe. Am I paranoid? Have *I* really made my son ill by excluding dairy products, soya, eggs, tomato, nuts, Trout, Kiwi fruit and all the other things I believe he's intolerant to? Am I harming my baby instead of helping him? Were the reactions he had a one off thing?

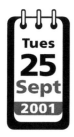 I leave the hospital with a churning feeling in my stomach and I doubt all I have done for my son. Maybe I should just calm down and leave everything in the hands of the Doctors; step back, take a deep breath and exhale.

On my way home I purchase the recommended rice pudding. When we get home I settle Jayden down and I do as the Doctor has told me. I put Jayden in his high chair in the living room, I feel apprehensive but here goes, I say a prayer and give him a tiny amount of his first taste of baby rice pudding. Oh my God!!! What is happening to my baby?!!! His mouth and face are swelling up in just a matter of seconds. I give him 5mls of Antihistamine, call an ambulance and explain what has happened, they arrive quickly. They examine my son and he is rushed to the hospital. Thank God he is stable and the swelling does not go to his throat.

I am so angry I want to scream at myself. I want to scream at the Doctors, "I TOLD YOU SO!"

Why did I listen to them? Why couldn't they have listened to me? They do not know my son like I do! I know what I see, I know what I feel. Just as I had expected, my baby had a major reaction to milk. He is allergic to dairy products. I am at the hospital and I am not happy. This is not a game! This is my son's life! Why is it so difficult for the Doctors to take my concerns seriously and work with me?

THIS WILL NOT HAPPEN AGAIN!

My earlier doubts fly away, I am doing the best for my son.

This is not my Fault

On our hospital admission, I was told that my son's deficiencies of Vitamin D, calcium and iron were due to me restricting his diet. I'm told over and over again that I need to take him off breast milk then he will eat better. However, I am convinced he won't be able to eat enough or eat a wide enough variety of foods right now so now is not the time. According to the 'The Red Book' he is underweight. He does not look underweight to me, 'The Red Book' is just a guideline. Jayden is fine. Mostly I'm upset with myself. I should have been more confident with my decision about him not eating dairy products! I want to shout at everyone and tell them to 'listen to me so I can help my son!'. I need to help my son - and we will NOT be put in this position again!

Exhale!

Back To Naturopathy

After the dairy product incident I contact Vanessa the Naturopathic Practitioner again and meet up with her. I explain to her what happened at the hospital. She tells me that because Jayden's Eczema is so severe, it would be difficult for him to absorb the nutrients he needs from food

– that includes the nutrients from my breast milk. She tells me about the role of sunlight, Vitamin D and the calcium connection. She goes on to explain that Eczema is a reflection of the digestive system – dry, flaky and leaky, so it wasn't my fault as the doctors suggested. She says his digestive system is probably immature and I should continue to breast feed him until I feel it is okay to take him off. She explains that calm, wet foods and a balanced diet will help Jayden immensely. 'Calming' foods are easy to digest foods - think creamy and soft rather than crunchy and rigid, they often contain calming nutrients that actually relax your nervous system and boost your mood.

Examples of some of the calm and wet foods we used: sweet potato, brown rice, broccoli, blueberry, avocado and oats. I also give Jayden Aloe Vera as an anti-inflammatory remedy, Camomile to drink and to bathe in to calm him and help reduce the itching. We are advised to avoid all foods that could absorb or take moisture away – wheat, salt and sugar being the three main culprits.

Additionally, processed foods are to be completely avoided while Omega oils 3, 6 and 9, lots of liquids, soups, and a calm stress-free environment are his prescription. She says it is a good idea to avoid all the common allergens and difficult to digest foods until he is at least three years old when his system will be stronger and more mature. Vanessa makes a lot of sense to me I begin on this course immediately. The diet changes will make my son more comfortable, however there seems to be no miracle cure.

Learning to cope with the condition

It is a fact that children living in England (or similar climates) with brown or dark skin are more prone to becoming deficient in Vitamin D, which can lead to Rickets and a variety of other ailments, there is extensive research available. Jayden was one of those statistics and he was further compromised because he was born in February – the winter season and the lack of London sunshine anyway! Even the little sun we had when it came out, couldn't get to him as so much of his skin would be covered because of the cold weather or bandaged for protection because of his Eczema. Lack of Vitamin D means the body cannot absorb Calcuim and other vital vitamins and minerals. Jayden didn't stand a chance.

IT WASN'T MY FAULT!!!

It would have been great to have been armed with this knowledge and start my baby on a course of Vitamin D much earlier on.

Knowledge is Key

O ne of the most overwhelming feelings for me was one of helplessness. I'm a person that always finds solutions to problems. When I discovered my son had Eczema and Allergies it didn't seem like a big deal because I was going to find the solution very quickly. How difficult could it be? I was traumatised by how difficult it actually was because I was looking for an instant cure.

It was the feeling of being out of control that propelled me to learn as much as I could about Eczema and Allergies. After all, wasn't I supposed to be the one to make my son better...?

I gathered information about what to do by observation, reading, from relatives, friends and strangers who would stop me in the street and give me advice, I didn't always need to ask. I tried some of the remedies, but nothing helped long-term, I thought that this was a problem. Today I understand that even short term remedies are good, I needed to celebrate the victory even if they were short lived.

I spent hours on the internet and with my head in books looking for help, alternatives, respite, hope, a light at the end of the tunnel – anything that would relieve my baby's discomfort. But as time went by I realised I couldn't cure Jayden. I felt so helpless and therefore worthless. I felt as if I was being punished for something I did wrong, but I didn't know what that could be. It was all so crushing. Of course now I know this wasn't true, but at the time I was stressed and not rational.

Eczema is a disease that is individual, therefore a remedy that works well for one sufferer may not help another. Sometimes I would find a new treatment and for a few days or even weeks there would be a big change. I would rejoice and shout out, "At last I've found the perfect remedy!" only to find out later that even perfect remedies become irritating after a while. However, giving up was not an option, I had to move on to find the next solution, this 'moving on' is necessary because of the nature of the disease.

I reviewed my son's diet, making sure it was rich in fish oils, omegas 3, 6 and 9 to ensure his bones stayed strong especially after the Rickets diagnosis. I found out about Oil of Evening Primrose and asked my Doctor if he would prescribe it, he agreed to trial Jayden on it for a few months. After the trial he said there was 'no marked improvement' so the prescription was withdrawn – I purchased it myself and continued. We added plenty of water to his diet, this cure, that cure ... I did this and not that... added this and took away that... always making adjustments and trying to make things perfect for him. I cried due to the absence of my mother, Lucy Charles whom I'd lost many years before my baby was born. She would have known what to do I thought. It was a lonely and difficult time.

Looking back, I was a wreck. When I was pregnant my plan was to go back to work when my baby was six months old, however, it didn't work out that way. I had no intention of paying someone to take care of my child whilst he had these conditions. No member of my family could take the job on – they were all busy with their own lives – but realistically, I wasn't going to leave him with anyone anyway, even if they were available. There was only one thing to do and that was for me to stay at home with my baby and take care of him full time.

This decision took a toll on my finances but I didn't know any other way, it had to be done. I 'maxed' out my credit cards and went into debt buying my son all the promises of a cure. I even purchased a battery operated contraption that promised to 'eliminate the itch'. It was called the 'Eletronic Itch Stopper'. I used it for around two months - it didn't work for us. Some people say they had great success with it. What else could I have done? I had to explore all the possibilities.

I joined the National Eczema Society. This organisation has lots of information about Eczema. I read the articles in their magazine looking for hope, it's informative, there's a help-line and there are lots of ideas.

A New-Found Confidence

I allowed some Health Professionals to make me feel insecure about how I cared for my baby, because they were concerned about the restrictions I had made to my son's diet. Looking back I can understand their concerns, but back then all I knew was, I was doing my best. I could have kicked myself for listening to a Doctor who insisted I give my baby dairy products. As a result Jayden had a severe allergic reaction. From then on, I decided that Doctors on the whole, go by a set of conventional rules about how to treat the condition, and those rules were not always the best for my son, because of the nature of the disease sufferers can react differently. I would treat my son together with them and not ignore my instincts. Of course I met many Doctors and Consultants who were very helpful, listened to my concerns, admitted when they did not know something and helped us the best they could.

Things feel very different today, we have moved back to Hackney and Jayden's GPs and Consultants listen and take on board our concerns and approaches. They understand how complicated it can be to treat Eczema and Allergies and how everyone responds uniquely to treatments. I need to continue to do my research and play the major part in my son's treatment, so I do.

The more things became difficult the more I did my research with greater vigour, confidence and intensity. With this new-found confidence, I would go to the Health Professionals knowing the facts (well, a little), and a list of what I needed. I would get the information I needed from them, look it up online and in books and then together with my own research, decide whether or not to use, or do what was prescribed or recommended, I called it team work.

When Jayden was younger his prescription was often for stronger and stronger Steroids and petroleum-based skin applications. This was not my idea of a solution, but it did have its' place in his treatment.

SMALL VICTORIES

Every moment of comfort for my baby was a victory. He could have a day when he didn't itch and his skin was comfortable and we would breathe a sigh of relief but the next day could be horrendous and it would be as if the Eczema and itching came out of nowhere!

The itching was the most difficult to manage. Many products claimed to be able to manage it, they obviously don't work for everyone and not a single one of them worked for my baby.

I would read the ingredients and side-effects of all medication before deciding whether to use it or ask for an alternative. I rejected products e.g. on the basis of them containing too much sugar because I was concerned about the large intake in his oral medication ruining his teeth before they even had the chance to emerge. On occasions I sensed my doctor was not happy with my requests. As I became more aware of what Jayden needed, I managed to convince my GP to prescribe, Propolis Cream and Aloe Vera. This helped me to feel in control, which was important to me. These were treatments to help strengthen my baby's immune system. He still uses these products today.

It was when Jayden was around 18 months that a friend introduced me to Aloe Vera juice. I gave my son 5mls every day. It tasted bitter, but I was confident that it would be good for him. When his skin was inflamed I would apply it to cotton wool and dab it on directly. It helped with inflammation. It has been consistent in Jayden's treatment and wellbeing. Overall, Aloe Vera has been our 'Piece de resistance'. Aloe Vera is also known as 'nature's gift' with a rich source of over two hundred naturally occurring nutritional substances.

The decision to do 'my thing' and go with my instincts was empowering, this was definitely a step in the right direction for me. I was happier and less stressed because I felt more in control, I needed that. I began to realise and accept that Eczema was a condition that needed to be managed, it couldn't be healed overnight, therefore the pressure I had created for myself – was lifted. With that new understanding, the task was different and felt more do-able, my job was to make as many moments as possible, as good as possible.

Battling Doctors

Following our consultations with Vanessa, our Naturo-pathic Practitioner, I understood that it is important to treat Eczema, Allergies and intolerances internally as well as externally. Skin applications were not the solution on their own – yes they could help to soothe and calm the skin and make it look better, but there was something happening inside that was causing Jayden's skin to flare up in the first place and this needed to be addressed.

My biggest issue with the treatment of Eczema was the actual skin moisturisers that had to, of course, be placed directly onto the skin. As with many sufferers, my son's skin was often cracked open, sensitive and sore therefore the moisturisers were quickly absorbed into his bloodstream, which couldn't be good if they were full of chemicals. I wanted the moisturisers to be as safe and as gentle as possible, the preparations needed to be low in chemical additives, but they weren't. I expressed my concerns to my GP and other Health Practitioners, but they had no satisfactory answers or alternatives for me. They said that the applications were all 'clinically tested', so they were safe. What else could they say?

I continually looked at improving my knowledge and boosting my son's immune system at the same time. I began to think that his Allergies and Eczema were there because of an underlying problem and that this underlying problem had predisposed him to Eczema and Allergies. As a child I suffered from Eczema and Jayden's father had Hay Fever, so Jayden had inherited that from us. However, I reasoned that if I could make him as strong as possible he could fight off whatever came his way and the condition would be less severe. Boosting his immune system was one of my priorities.

In my research I came across an article published by Pierre Fabre Research Institute, entitled, 'Low-Salt Water Reduces Intestinal Permeability in Atopic Patients'. This study further confirmed what my Naturopath, Vanessa had told me, Eczema needed to be treated on the inside as well as outside. I booked an appointment to speak to our GP about the article, he admitted he had never heard of this so I sent him the link to the study.

THE LOW-SALT WATER STUDY
This study found clinical evidence that the water at Avène Spa in France helped patients with atopic skin conditions. By drinking the water, patients' skins showed improvement as the water got to work healing the permeability in their intestines.

Bandaging Systems

Some days parts of Jayden's body would be stuck to his clothing or bed sheets. I would have to run a warm bath and soak him in it until they came away from him. Other times when I would remove his clothes I could see and hear the tiny particles of his skin falling to the surface. It was surreal.

From the age of one until Jayden was around 3 years old, I put bandages to protect his skin from his scratching, stop infection and keep moisture in. Although the bandages were benficial for these reasons they generated heat - the term Eczema is derived from the Greek meaning to 'boil out' - wrapping therefore had its disadvantages.

Itchoplast was one of the best bandaging systems I used for Jayden. It was packed with a creamy substance containing zinc. When I removed these bandages from his legs and arms, his skin would be well moisturised and soft. Itchoplast bandages were definitely great for the condition, but he hated having them on. He just wanted to have his legs and arms out in the open so when I put them on, his mission was to get them off.

After about a year I stopped using these Itchoplast bandages when I noticed he had developed small black and white patches at the front of one ankle. I put it down to the substances in the bandages, as this was listed as one of the possible side effects.

Tubifast has a range of leggings, vests and tube shaped bandages that I would dampen and apply to Jayden's heavily moisturised body, legs and arms. This would keep his skin cool, moist and supple for a while. As Jayden got older he became a master at getting out of these. At two years old he could verbally express his dislike of having his body wrapped, "I want no clothes on!" He used to cry and run away from me when I got the bandages out. That was a testing time, I felt sad for him, but I needed to do it. We played different games and sang songs when putting them on but he still hated having them on – Now at the age of 13, he says he still remembers that time.

He didn't like having to put clothes on, he wanted to be able to get to his skin without having to manoeuvre through clothing. Often it was impossible to allow his skin to be uncovered for long periods of time because it was so sore, the very act of the air passing his skin would trigger the itch and make him scratch himself into a frenzy. I can still see that deep concentration on his face as he got to the itch. It was almost as if he was in a trance. He couldn't hear my pleas for him to, "Tap your skin baby" or "let mummy do it".

The scratching is so damaging, much more so than the Eczema itself.

His wish came true when he was around six years old, we agreed, as long as I filed down his fingernails and toenails every day, he could sleep without any clothes, on occasion.

Help is at Hand

Another difficult thing to deal with was the judgment other people passed on me due to Jayden's condition. I remember one particular afternoon in the lovely July sunshine, Jayden and I were on the last leg of our journey home from Southend-on-Sea with some friends. We board-

> Scratching technique taught at Avène Spa. I would slide the back of my fingernails along Jayden's skin and flick outwards as my palms open up. In this way the scratching action would not damage his skin.

ed a bus for our final ten-minute journey. Jayden was tired and itchy and it got worse whilst we were on the bus. I was distracting him the best I could, playing 'Peek-a-Boo' and performing a puppet show with his teddy. He began crying because he wanted to scratch himself and was frantically trying to get at his legs. I was saying, "Let mummy do it" and scratching his legs with my fingernails in a backwards technique taught at Avène Spa. However, this wasn't relieving the itch, so he wanted to do it himself. Eventually, I let him and helped where I could.

At that point a woman's voice came from the back of the bus saying, "Why doesn't she take care of that baby properly?"

I assumed she was talking about me. I never looked up. It was easier to pretend I didn't hear her, but I wanted to explain to her how much I do take care of my son and I was taking care of him right now. I wanted her to know everything. I wanted her to understand what she was seeing. However I found no words, I simply left the bus at the very next stop and walked the rest of the way home in tears.

So many times we only see a snapshot of a moment in someone's life: We see them in passing; in the street; in a shop; wherever – and we make judgements. I'm so aware of this today. Although I know I judge automatically, like most human beings, I try to remember that incident to stop me in my tracks and make me rethink.

Peer Support

By the time Jayden was 18 months old I decided that I needed to set up a group to help parents with children with Eczema and Allergies. I realised that if I was struggling, then many more people had to be in the same position. I joined a course in Newham, East London, for parents wanting to start various self-help groups. The lady running the course was called Alison – she was a great motivation and inspiration. She had two young sons who were both Autistic. They had inspired her to set up various groups, write a book about Autism and run workshops, she was amazing and resourceful. She cared and I am eternally grateful to her, for her role in my life.

The people on the course were all parents of children with what I would call major disabilities (compared to me) – Cerebral Palsy, Autism and wheelchair bound. The parents talked about having their homes converted to be fully accessible, having to clean excretion from the walls, making their homes safe for their child who had gone on to develop Epilepsy.

During the first week my question was, what did I really have to complain about? My child has severe Eczema, Allergies and intolerances, their children didn't have the hope of growing out of their conditions, they were simply coping the best they could with the problems they had and looking for solutions to help them cope. What am I doing here? I questioned myself and my ability to be a capable mother.

I felt like a fake being there and asking for help. After the first session, I explained this to the group, they were supportive and assured me that I had every right to be with them and they welcomed me. After a few weeks I felt part of the group, supported and understood, I looked forward to our weekly meetings. Eventually

I set up a phone support group for parents of children with Eczema and Allergies.

Disability Living Allowance (DLA)

Alison, the lady running the course, told me about Disability Living Allowance (DLA), which I had never heard about. She explained that it was an Allowance to help parents and carers and the disabled person live better lives. The Allowance could help me with Jayden's special diet, clothing, travelling and respite. My life with my son was extraordinary – I would wake up eight times a night and all through the day I attended to my son, always on the lookout for allergens wherever we went. There was no rest for us. Alison advised me to apply for it.

I delayed applying for the DLA for weeks – I didn't think I could get it, there were people in far worse situations than Jayden and I. Alison was convinced I had a good case and encouraged me to proceed. Reluctantly, I sent for the form and when it finally arrived it took me a few emotional days to complete it. I cried as I documented for the first time, what it was like taking care of my son. Putting our lives into words, down on paper, made me feel really sad for my baby. I posted the form and didn't expect to get anything back.

On 15th April 2004, 7 weeks after filling out the form, I received a letter from the Department for Work and Pensions which said, "We confirm that you have been awarded Disability Living Allowance for help with personal care at the highest rate." I really could not believe it – God knows this was a breakthrough. At times I really thought that I had lost my mind because I was feeling so stressed over my baby's condition when I thought I should have been able to 'get on with it', after all there were millions of people in worse situations. But now it was official – how we were living was distressing and we were entitled to financial support! I cried a lot that day. From that day I gave myself a 'little break' as they say. It was okay to feel overwhelmed because my situation was officially 'overwhelming'.

> To claim DLA In England and Wales, get in touch with your Department of Social Security, they should be able to help you. I don't know what's on offer in other areas or countries but it is worthwhile doing some research and contacting charities and Social Services who should be able to point you in the right direction.

Financially things changed from that day and we were able to live a little easier. I would get taxis more often instead of struggling on public transport with an uncomfortable child, I could buy better quality, pure cotton clothing, special clothes to protect Jayden's body from him scratching. I could buy organic food all the time, which was three times more expensive than non-organic. I continued to try other products that promised to make him better, including Aloe Vera drink, Propolis Cream, and Aloe Vera Gelly – all this I could now afford.

After receiving the DLA, whenever I saw parents in the street, or at different functions with children scratching or children with obvious Eczema, I would tell them about the Allowance. Not one person I spoke to had heard about it, neither did they think they would be entitled to such financial help. I met with them to help fill out their forms if they wanted, or we would talk about what we had done and what we were doing to help our children. We went over what worked and what didn't, many contacted me later with the news that they had been given some financial assistance. It felt satisfying to help others even if it was just a little.

I spoke to my GP about the DLA and gave him the information so he could advise patients who might be eligible for it, he hadn't heard of it either!

Letting Go

Unsurprisingly, my baby and I were inseparable in his early years. However, when he was 20 months old, I booked myself on a two day conference which promised to teach me how to make a lot of money quickly. The thought of being financially free and able to give my son the best of everything was attractive, so I decided to go.

I arranged for a friend to take care of my son. This was the very first time leaving him. I prepared a list of what needed to be done and when to do it, to take care of my baby and I left. The two days away were great. I thought about Jayden constantly but I was given clear instructions by my friend to only call twice a day. She had decided that I needed a break. At the end of the conference I rushed back to collect my son. He was distressed – his skin hadn't been moisturised enough (every twenty minutes was what was needed) and he had lots of small cuts where he had been able to get to his skin and scratch for hours it seemed.

I was so angry, not at my dear friend – she did her best – but at myself. Jayden's care was a full time job and she had a young son to take care of herself so I should have known it wouldn't have worked out well. It wasn't until he was three and a half years old that I would be able to gather up enough courage to let someone else take care of him and this was when he joined a nursery.

Rejection from Nurseries

When Jayden was three years old I began the process of finding a nursery for him. It was difficult for me to make this decision as he had hardly been out of my sight, but of course it was necessary.

I approached five nurseries in total. They were all happy to show us around and tell me why I should choose their nursery. However, when it came to me filling out the forms and being interviewed about Jayden and the special care he would need, because of his Allergies and Eczema, three of them said they couldn't risk having him at their nursery. It would mean they would have to make so many changes when it came to eating – they would have to check what food they supplied, check that the other children had washed their hands after dinner, so as not to possibly contaminate Jayden, maybe not allow certain foods in the nursery, train their staff and so on. It was just going to be too difficult, so they rejected my son.

This alarmed me. At the time I thought they wouldn't have my little boy in their nursery because they were too 'lazy' to make some changes?!!! I believed what they were doing was illegal but I had no strength to pursue this. I felt heartbroken and I cried. What about all those children with other disabilities that were obvious to see? What an injustice they would have to live with! It was a horrible feeling.

Today I wish I could remember the names of those nurseries, I wonder if they have changed their policies? I hope so.

The other two nurseries were more willing, but didn't have any money in their budget to send their staff for training, they said he couldn't join. Excuse? I don't know for sure.

Finally, I rang the Department of Education at Newham Council where we lived and spoke to a woman about my difficulties finding a nursery to accept my son. She sympathised with me and put me in touch with St Matthew's Nursery in East London. I went to meet the staff a few days later I loved it there and a short while later Jayden joined. They made all the necessary changes and welcomed Jayden with open arms. All I needed to do was supply my son's food.

The children now had to wash their hands very well, after eating as well as before, incase they ate something Jayden was allergic to. The staff moisturised my son's arms, hands, legs and feet every 30 minutes and more if he needed it. I trained them on using the Epipen and they later went on to have professional training. They were excellently accommodating!

Anxious To Let Go

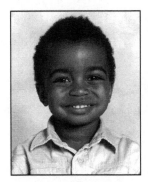 Jayden joining the nursery was a big step for us. It was a huge step for me. I had to learn to let go and feel comfortable and confident enough for someone else to take care of him. The first two weeks I had to stay on the premises, but out of sight, for any emergencies or queries. Jayden cried a lot the first and second day, but then he began to settle down and make friends. I brought lots of things in with me to keep me busy whilst I stayed out of sight, however I struggled to concentrate on what I had to do because I wanted to peek all the time to see how he was doing, what he was doing, who was near him etc. Eventually I learnt to leave him in their care.

The staff at the nursery were fantastic. Trust and confidence quickly built up between us and my son had a great time there. Nursery was two-and-a-half days a week. This gave me a little time to stop, sit down and have some time to myself. I used the time to catch up with housework, prepare food, shop and research. Sometimes I would just sleep the time away. The time passed by quickly. St Matthew's Nursery was a Godsend.

Sleep Deprivation

Not having enough sleep was one of the things that took its toll on me. In actual fact, it nearly threw me 'off the edge'. For the majority of the time, Jayden slept only forty-five minutes at a time. Very occasionally, it would be a short while before he went back to sleep (twenty to forty minutes), but most of the time he would take a a couple of hours to go back to sleep. Waking up all through the night became the norm. He would be scratching, crying, frustrated and so very uncomfortable. I would wash him, reapply creams, moisturisers, apply and reapply bandages and mittens that he had managed to take off. I would give him juices, water, breast milk, put 'Winnie the Pooh' video tapes on to distract him, hold his hands away from his body, play games to take his mind off his itching, and to stop him rubbing and scratching. Finally, I would put him back to sleep on my breast.

Sometimes I'd stand for hours with him in front of the fan trying to cool him down whilst the video of 'Winnie the Pooh' was running to distract him from his discomfort. I had to keep the heating off all the time and have the windows open so my son could stay cool. Even in the winter he would be hot – I would have to put on several layers of clothes to keep myself warm.

On other occasions in the early hours of the morning or late at night I'd go out into the street and walk up and down with him until he slept, cooled down or both. Sometimes I would put him in his buggy and push him around after doing all the other things, what else could I do? Eventually he would fall asleep and forty-five minutes later he would wake up and I'd do the same thing - all over again.

I got desperate and depressed, I cried every day because I couldn't make him better - that was what a mum was supposed to do. He was supposed to be enjoying his life and I was supposed to be enjoying him much more. Instead it was a battle of getting through each hour, each night, each day, each week. I felt unable to cope but I got on with it, not telling anyone how bad I felt.

On 29th August 2002, at the age of 18 months Jayden was prescribed Vallergan by his GP. This medication was to help calm him and aid him to sleep, so I could also sleep. I had my reservations and it took me several days to give it to him, but finally I did. The medicine had a terrible effect on him. Yes, it successfully put him to sleep but, he struggled in this drug induced state. He still scratched his skin, cried and tossed about, all with his eyes closed. It was like looking at him having a nightmare that I couldn't wake him from. What had I done? I felt so guilty. It was because I wanted us to sleep that

I had agreed to this medication. Needless to say I never gave it to him again.

There had to be another way, other ways! I continued to research to find more answers. What he needed was something to stop him from itching, so he wouldn't scratch – this was what was disturbing him and damaging his skin and ultimately not allowing him to rest. What we needed was help and sleep was the help we were crying out for and this eventually came about a year later when we took a trip to Avène in France.

Finding Relief in France – Avène Health Spa

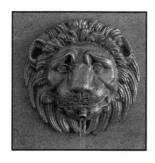One day in August 2003 I was surfing the internet for more information about Eczema and Allergies and came across a story about a woman who had a son with the same conditions as mine. Her description of the lack of sleep, sore skin, Allergies, helplessness, loneliness and isolation that she constantly faced, was so familiar, she could have been me.

This woman wrote how she had taken her son to a Spa in Avène, France, and had great success. Her son was not cured, but he was better than he had been before. He was more comfortable and happier and therefore, there was a significant improvement in the quality of their lives.

I researched Avène and found out that it was a Thermal Spa which first opened in 1786 in Southern France, two hour's drive from Montpellier. It is located in the Mountains, away from all the hassle of everyday life. It was somewhere to go and relax and heal while taking in the fresh air and healing waters. A place where 2,500 people visit each year for three weeks of treatment for various skin problems including: Eczema, psoriasis, burns and severe acne.

I contacted the Spa Centre and spoke to the Marie-Ange Martincic, the Director. She was reassuring and welcoming, I was convinced I needed to take Jayden there.

I booked our flights, accommodation and the recommended three weeks of treatment. There was so much to do. Jayden was drinking a litre of Oatly Drink (an alternative to milk) daily, I had carried out some investigations and found out I couldn't purchase it in France, so I ordered 21 litres of it and arranged with the management in Avène to have them delivered there. I packed a further 4 cartons in my luggage incase my order was delayed. Within three weeks of reading the article, Jayden and I arrived in France.

> Oatly Drink is a calcium-enriched alternative to milk, which contains an oat base (water, oats), rapeseed oil, salt, vitamins (D2, riboflavin, folic acid and B12), and calcium.

On arrival, we went straight to our apartment which was a bedsit and part of the Spa complex. The apartment had a bunk bed and a double bed. We both slept in the double bed. Jayden used the bunk bed as his castle. There was a bathroom with a shower attachment in the bath. Jayden used this space as his play house and would invite me over for tea and cake. There was a two-plate stove and a place to prepare food, a small cupboard for our food shopping, a dining table inside and a smaller table outside on the balcony where we ate. The bedsit was cosy, we felt safe and comfortable there.

The bedsit was situated on the third floor without a lift, but we managed. It was less than five minutes walk from the Spa. After unpacking our suitcases and having something to eat. I called a taxi and we went to the nearby town and purchased food for the week then got a taxi back to our bedsit.

Later that evening we were called to the small office in the apartment complex to meet the Doctor. He examined Jayden and prescribed the treatment for his three-week stay. Treatment would take place six days a week. There would be no treatments on Sundays – today.

Treatment Begins

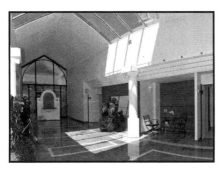

The morning after we arrived, the treatment started. It's Monday morning and we leave our apartment half an hour before our appointment.

I carry Jayden's buggy down the three flights of stairs and he walks down holding my hand. After a short walk we arrive at the Spa at 10am. There are people there from all over the world – Australians, Japanese, New Zealanders, Americans, Polish, Italians and French to name a few.

We go to the Reception and check-in. Here we are given bathrobes, slippers and 2 empty bottles to fill up with the water to drink during our treatment. These we keep until the end of the three weeks. From here we go to the changing rooms, undress and put on the bathrobes and slippers. Jayden wears swimming trunks under his bathrobe, I wear a swimsuit. I won't be having the treatment, but I will be getting wet and holding him in the showers if necessary.

The first part of the treatment is a jet spray directed onto the thickened parts of Jayden's skin – his knees, elbows, ankles and hands. He screams and protests a little every time it touches his body. However, the practitioner administering the treatment is very understanding and gentle with Jayden so it doesn't take him long to settle. It was to take him two weeks to get totally comfortable with this treatment and I did think of stopping it after the first session, but I was advised that the benefits were exceptional as it would help to stimulate the moisture in those thickened parts of Jayden's skin.

The second step of the treatment is a fifteen-minute massage. Jayden is placed on a plastic table which has lots of holes below for the water to escape through and a shower attachments above it. The masseuse wets my son's skin and massages all the thickened parts. Jayden frowns and cries a little as he stretches his arms out towards me so I can lift him off. I reassure him that it's ok to stay. It is all new to him, he only wants me to be near him and he certainly doesn't want some stranger massaging his sore skin with cool water. The masseuse is very good with him and slowly wins his confidence, about a week later Jayden settles down. My job is to distract him by singing, telling stories and making funny faces at him. The distraction works, I am good at it, I have had lots of practice!

Following this massage is a 20 minute Jacuzzi. Jayden is put in a large bath, where the jets of water massage and stimulate his skin. There are around five baths in this room with a child in each and a parent sitting beside the bath with the job of supervising and entertaining their child, or convincing them it is okay and there isn't anything to be afraid of. Other parents can sit and read as it's their third week or their third year at the Spa and their child is accustomed to the treatment. The children are given lots of toys to play with in the bath which is great. Jayden has his Smurf and his wind-up Diver in the bath with him. After getting used to the vigorous bubbling of the Jacuzzi, he enjoys this bath. However every time the water splashes his face he gets up and looks startled. It takes him a while to accept the splashing in his face but he doesn't like it one bit.

For the next treatment, he is wrapped in his thick white robe and taken to the play room to rest. Once we get there he plays quietly for twenty minutes. After this we are directed to another room with lots of books and more toys. I read Jayden stories as we lounge in the chairs. In this room his hands, ankles, feet and knees are wrapped in gauze and saturated with the Spa water. It is my job to keep these hydrated over the next twenty minutes with a spray bottle filled with Spa water.

Finally, we are led to a shower cubicle where soft jets of water from around a dozen nozzles are directed at him from all angles. He is only tiny so I go into the cubicle with him and hold him on my hip for the whole session because he doesn't enjoy the water spraying on his face. We sing and play as the therapist outside the cubicle adjusts the jets of water to the prescribed pressures and vapours. The session ends with a fine mist coming out at us. I believe that this was to massage and penetrate the skin, thereby hydrating and stimulating his skin. The whole session lasts around two hours.

After his first session Jayden's skin feels softer, I feel hopeful and Jayden seems happy. Everything else is the same, he still scratches and cries and wakes often during that night. I am not concerned because I am aware that things will need time to adjust and we were told that we wouldn't see an immediate improvement, I know that much by now. We were given water bottles at the start of the treatment and encouraged to drink during our treatment and throughout our stay. The water heals on the inside as well as the outside. We fill our bottles up from the fountain at the Spa and carry them back to our apartment to use for drinking and cooking. I am confident the water, fresh air, fresh food and relaxation will all contribute to his healing. During the course of the day we go back to the Spa with more bottles for filling because we use the water for everything at the apartment.

A Relaxing Environment

The days and nights felt long at Avène. The treatment lasted a couple of hours then we had the rest of the day to ourselves. The centre had a variety of workshops to educate and further help us in our battles – how to scratch the skin without damaging it is one of the things that has stuck in my memory. It was so different from being at home, I compare it to a therapeutic holiday.

Once a week we would go shopping in a large town close to Avène. We would catch a taxi down the mountain, along a narrow winding road. This journey took about 45 minutes. In between doing our weekly shop we would visit the local village for fresh meat and vegetables. There were also 'shop vans' that would visit the Spa village, there was a Bakery, a Butcher and a Grocer. It was so different and lovely, we found it easy to chill out there. The whole experience helped us to de-stress which added to the successful outcome of the treatment.

After Jayden's treatments we visited other families, we rested, played in the park, played mini golf and walked along the country lanes looking at beautiful flowers, herbs and wildlife. My son learned to recognise Rosemary, Lavender and Peppermint plants as they were everywhere on our walks. We picked them and used the Rosemary in our cooking. I made tea with the Peppermint and Jayden would eat the leaves we picked and call them his sweets. The Lavender we put on our pillows in socks. All these herbs contributed to our relaxing stay.

In the early evenings we play our version of snooker back at Hotel Val d'Orb which is attached to the Spa. Of course I have to let him win...

Avène is a peaceful, fun and healing place to be.

Avène Duck go Aawk Aawk

In the play park I sit on the swing with Jayden on my lap and we sing 'Row, row, row your boat...' He sits on the wooden horse near to the stream, climbs the wooden frame and goes up and down the slide. He has so much fun here.

Along our way to or from the play park we bounce pebbles on the stream which is just outside our apartment. Jayden loves this game, we still play it today. We stay by the stream for hours.

From our apartment we can hear the ducks throughout the day. Today Jayden asks, "Mummy what's that noise?" I tell him it's the ducks. He looks at me and frowns. We go down to the stream where there are lots of ducks, some are walking on the banks quite close to us and the ducklings follow their mummies. We watch for

Keen learner
Jayden hadn't started nursery at this time but I would take him to our local 'Parent and Baby Group' once a week where they would tell stories and do other activities. He was a keen learner. I read to him almost every single day, even through what was going on.

a while then Jayden just stares and frowns at them and then says with a gasp:

"Ah, mummy they made a mistake!"

"Who made a mistake, darling?"

"Nursery and the books," he replied urgently.

"What did they do, baby?"

"Mummy, ducks don't go 'quack, quack', ducks go aawk, aawk!"

He covers his mouth as he continuously shakes his head saying, "Ohhh noooooo!" He had learned the French word for duck and starts saying, "Les Canards go aawk aawk".

I pick him up and can't stop laughing. My little boy is so clever, so observant, and he's right – the sound the ducks made was 'aawk aawk', not 'quack quack'!

Learning French

In order for us to shop safely, I bought a 'French-to-English' dictionary to help with translating the words on food packaging. However, there were many words we couldn't find in the dictionary so we had to ask the staff and people along the way to translate for us. During this process, Jayden learned to identify all of the French words on the packages that he was allergic to like eggs (oeufs), milk (lait) and nuts (noix). He would read the packages and

> Over the years I did get much better with my cooking and baking, I'm pretty good now – Jayden thinks so too!

together we would make the decision as to what we could and couldn't buy. He became an expert. When he didn't find the allergens on the packages, he would shout, "I CAN HAVE THIS, MUMMY!" and put it in our basket.

Often, when he couldn't have something he wanted, we made it. For example, we made our own milkshakes using Oatly Drink to replace milk and we added fruit and a little sugar. It was fun but sometimes frustrating for both of us. Occasionally Jayden would get upset that he couldn't have what was on the shelf in the supermarket and my attempts at creating something similar were not always great. However, he was always pleased with my efforts.

Until Jayden was seven years old, it wasn't a big deal to him that he couldn't eat certain foods. However, from then he began to realise his restrictions in a different way and sometimes became upset. Today he fully understands his restrictions and what they mean and he isn't happy with them, however he gets on with it and every day we look towards a future without Allergies.

I have had to be on my toes and find alternatives, I have dozens now – we make great cakes, biscuits, chocolate bars, frothy bedtime hot chocolate, doughnuts and much more – but that's another book!

Incident at the Spa

Although things were mostly good at Avène, we had a few frustrating times too. One day, just after finishing treatment at the Spa, Jayden was sitting happily in his buggy leafing through a newspaper that I had let him have from the reception. We were on our way to the local village and then suddenly he started scratching his hands frantically. I quickly guessed he was having a reaction from the ink on the newspaper, this was a new reaction!

I took him out of his buggy and rushed back to the Spa into the restroom and ran his hands under the water. By this time they were swollen, he was irritated, upset and very uncomfortable. He began to cry then scream and bite his little hands for relief from the itching. I gave him 5mls of Antihistamine, held him to comfort him the best I could. He wanted to be left alone to scratch his hands and I was in his way. It looked like he wanted to tear his little hands off. I sat on the floor in the restroom and just cried with him. I kept saying, 'Sorry baby, I'm so sorry." There was nothing else I could do. Through his tears he wept the words, "sorry mummy, don't cry", and he hugged me". My crying was upsetting him but I couldn't stop. I held him tight and told him there was nothing to be sorry about. That was a moment I felt as if I just couldn't cope. After about thirty minutes the symptoms calmed down. He was exhausted and fell asleep. We went straight back to our apartment, we could go to the village another day.

We Were Not Alone

My son was two and half years old and it had taken up until now to find this 'help' – or rather, this long to find an organisation that thoroughly understood us and actually helped in the way we needed.

We went to the Spa at the same time each day and got to know a few other families who we spent time with during our stay outside of treatment times. We met parents who had the same history as us. Our children had Eczema and similar Allergies, food intolerances, itching and scratching patterns. We were comfortable in each others' company. We had food we could share with each other, (that was a first for us). Our children played, got itchy and scratched together, then played some more. No one looked odd or out of place, there wasn't a problem – we were in the same boat, a family, it was really nice.

One morning, I met a woman in the changing rooms at the Spa, she was sitting on the bench crying whilst her baby scratched frantically, besides her. She had put on the moisturisers and done all she knew to help her child, however her child was now in that scratching, 'trance zone' (my definition) she looked totally exhausted and broken. Words were not needed. We didn't even speak the same language. I held her and she sobbed, I shed tears with her, she appreciated that I knew what she was feeling. After a few minutes we parted, smiled and continued to get our children ready for their treatments.

Everyday parents would share stories of their own battles with Eczema and Allergies. Listening to their stories was like listening to myself, we were bonded by our common journeys with our children. We shared stories, recipes, solutions and talked about how we dealt with the peculiarities of our children's predicaments. We laughed and cried together. It was incredibly empowering and those experiences I draw strength from even today, ten years later.

Sleep

After 10 days of treatment at Avène, Jayden slept for TEN HOURS! This was a massive breakthrough! I kept waking up and looking at him to check that he was okay. I had gotten into the habit of waking up without being woken by him. This sleep routine continued for much of the remainder of our stay. The Eczema was still very much there, but it was less, the itching was less so the scratching was less, therefore the stress was less, so everything was so much calmer and easier to cope with. By the end of our three weeks, we were like two different people. Jayden was more comfortable and less stressed, I was less stressed and this had a positive effect on him.

Preparing to go Home

I wanted to live and work at the Spa forever. I felt afraid to leave Avène because I knew that when we got home and things went back to normal the Eczema would get bad again. The staff were supportive and the treatment was excellent. It wasn't excellent because the Eczema was less, it was excellent because the staff at Avène understood Eczema and Allergies, they understood the peculiarities of it and how individual it was. They understood the emotional and physical aspect of it. They listened and gave treatment and advice based on each person. It was a breath of fresh air. Here, I was not seen as a nuisance mum, I was simply 'rightly concerned' and searching proactively for answers to support the wellbeing of my son. I was an excellent mum.

On our departure we were given a bag of lotions, creams, Spa water in a spray canister, and a wealth of knowledge, information and techniques so we were prepared and better armed to cope at home. We were also given a beautiful Avène robe, a video about the Spa, a heartfelt hug and sent off with best wishes. What a haven! I wanted to take home litres of the Spa water but managed only four.

Major Turning Point

Our stay at Avène was a major turning point in our lives and really equipped us to deal with Eczema and Allergies in a better way. If I had known about this place when Jayden was younger, I'm sure our journey would not have been so traumatic. However, I believe everything happens at the right time and I thank God I found the Spa when I did.

Coming home, things did get bad again, but slowly. However, because we had learned so much and had a range of different techniques to help us cope, things were no longer such a nightmare for me. Jayden didn't know anything different but because I was calmer, things were just better for him. We were advised to have three weeks of treatment for the next three years. So we did, and it definitely helped. We visited Avène again the following year when Jayden was three and half years old and then once more when he was five and a half. Even now after many years, we have fond memories and we are still in contact with them.

Avène highlighted the importance of staying hydrated inside and out. Before I even knew the significance of water and Eczema, I noticed that my son always wanted to drink. At eighteen months old, after I stopped breastfeeding, he would drink almost two litres of liquid each day – he was a thirsty baby! Research shows that people with Eczema need more hydrating than those without it.

The good news is treatment at Avène is available on the NHS so ask your GP about it. If he/she doesn't know about it, look it up on the NHS website.

Lies, Deceit and the 'Miracle Cure'

Along our journey we came across many companies which made massive claims and promises to cure Eczema. I purchased lotions, creams, bath additives, contraptions and various therapies in stores and over the web, but they didn't work. It didn't enter my mind for a moment that I might be being conned - because I believed (and still do) Eczema was so individual, the products just didn't work for my son. The sellers may have had an ulterior motive to lie and play on my desperation in a bid to make money, but the products did no obvious harm to my son, so I didn't suspect anything malicious...

Until...

...One day I came across a product with the promise of 'completely healing Eczema in a matter of days'. This was to change my mind.

'Wau Wau' Cream

In October 2001 when Jayden was just 8 months old, I spoke to a lady I met over the internet and she told me about this 'revolutionary' cream she had used on her baby girl and it had taken her Eczema away completely.

I asked her what was in it. She said it was a totally natural product – containing the root of the Yam plant and a 'Wau Wau' plant. I had heard of Yam, but not the 'Wau Wau' plant, however that didn't matter. She said neither had she before she was introduced to the product. The product was from Ghana. I had always thought there must be so many cures around the world for so many diseases that we may never get to hear about, so why not this one? The cream was sold as 100% natural and satisfaction guaranteed – I was impressed and excited. She put me in contact with a man called Alan.

I quickly contacted Alan and was anxious to meet him that same day but he wasn't available, so the next day I met him in North London and paid him £30 in cash for the 250 gram jar of cream. I asked him why, if this cream was so good, it wasn't being sold to Pharmacists. He said something along the lines of it being a conspiracy and pharmaceutical companies not wanting to lose all the money they made from Eczema sufferers. 'Wau Wau' cream would put an end to the multi-billion pound Eczema treatment market," he said. "It's political."

I thanked him and went home. That same evening I decided to do a Patch Test on my son. I was supposed to carry out this Test over 5 days to make sure that there were no adverse reactions, but, I couldn't wait. I was sure it would be fine. I was too excited, or should I say impatient and desperate for something to work! I said a prayer, put the 'Wau Wau' cream on a small area of Jayden's arm and waited four hours. Everything seemed fine, so I put the cream all over one of Jayden's arms and waited until the morning to see the effects.

We Have Found a Cure!

In the morning I saw that the cream had already made his arm comfortable. Before my eyes the inflammation had gone down. His arm looked better than any product had ever made it look, that was all I needed to see. I confidently applied the cream everywhere else the Eczema was, including his eyelids, because 'it was safe' – Alan and the lady using it on her child had said so. Jayden seemed to sigh with relief as his skin calmed down very quickly. This is it! I laughed and danced for joy, at last we had found a cure! Jayden was going to be okay now, no more suffering! I rejoiced and started looking forward to Jayden's total healing. This 'Wau Wau' cream was something I needed to share with the world!

Three days later it was Sunday and we went to church as usual. My friends there knew about our battle, I got up and gave a testimony about the amazing 'Wau Wau' cream. People came to see me afterwards to get more information. It seemed everyone had a use for it.

I had planned to go to my GP and tell him to recommend it to all his patients with Eczema and end their nightmares too! How come this was kept secret? Why didn't the manufacturers just sell the cream to a pharmaceutical company and go through the proper channels? Maybe they could set up a movement or something and let all parents and carers of Eczema sufferers protest in support. This could literally help millions of people! I was very excited.

I couldn't understand why Alan met me so secretly, however, I reassured my doubts by reminding myself of the explanation he had given me – "it's political". We met up a few more times and as Jayden continued to progress, I would take orders for friends.

A little while later Jayden had an appointment at St John's Hospital Institute of Dermatology in South London. He had been using the 'Wau Wau' cream now for about two months. In the waiting room I told parents about the cream. Some were sceptical and didn't want any information, others gave me their telephone numbers and we spoke later.

Doubts and Suspicion

I told the Consultant about this amazing cream. 'The past two month have been a breakthrough', I said. He was unmoved by my news and said that the cream was probably full of Steroids and I should be careful. I never thought for a moment that the cream could be harmful. I protested, 'the cream is labelled natural, and my son's skin looks better'. He smiled and said 'natural' doesn't mean it is safe, he said they could check it out at the hospital lab if I brought in a sample, I agreed to do so.

A week later, the skin on my hands began to feel stiff and dried out. Yes, I did wash my hands constantly because I wanted to make sure that I didn't pass infection on to my son's broken skin, but this was a different feeling. I began to suspect that maybe the cream did have something harsh in it, something else that was not identified and now causing a problem to my skin.

I decided that I would take the cream to the hospital lab to be analysed the next day. I called the lab to ask where I should bring the sample and they said that they had already analysed several jars of 'Wau Wau' cream and they were full of Steroids as they suspected. It was dangerous to use because each jar contained different amounts of Steroid so you had no idea what amounts the body was absorbing. They also said the creams were not mixed well either and there were lumps of Steroids in it.

I was shocked and angry. Was this true or was it a conspiracy? I asked the Technician many questions: Was he sure? Was it the same 'Wau Wau' cream I was using? How did he get hold of it? I put down the phone and was incandescent with rage. How can people be so greedy and wicked just to make a few bucks?! I called Alan and told him about my conversation with the Lab Technician at the hospital. "Is the cream helping your son?" he asked. "Yes it is," I said. "Well then, you should ignore this report!" He's right, I thought. I can't vent my anger at him anyway, he is not the manufacturer of the product, just a distributor. Is any of this even true? I stopped using the product as I no longer felt confident.

Suspicion Confirmed

Soon after I switched on the TV and there was a documentary investigating 'Wau Wau' cream! It turned out that this cream had been banned previously, but it was still being sold illegally. It was imported from Ghana and had unsolicited amounts of Steroids in it – the authorities tested many jars and the amount of Steroid in each jar varied, just as the Lab Technician had said.

As I watched, I heard parents talking about how brilliant the cream was at first and then how adversely their child's skin had been affected once they stopped. I felt sick to my stomach. I had been putting this cream on my son's eyelids!!! I prayed that Jayden would not be adversely affected because I knew that Steroids could thin the skin, I thank God he wasn't! I had stopped using the 'Wau Wau' cream and 48 hours later the Eczema came back with vengence. I had to contact all the people I had introduced to the cream and ask them to also tell the people they told about the cream. Luckily they were understanding. To this day the skin on my right hand, the hand I used to apply the cream to Jayden, feels slightly hardened.

Beware of Con Artists

As you can see, through my desperation I got caught up in the world of con artists. I spent a lot of time and thousands of pounds over the internet and various outlets buying promises, remedies – natural creams, lotions, potions, bath additives, bed sheets, sleep wear, anti-itch contraptions, you name it, I bought it! I even visited different Natural Health Professionals, sometimes travelling hours to get to them. Many people are out there looking to get rich off someone else's pain and desperation. I had a cupboard full of products that didn't work, thousands of pounds worth of promises, piled high!

The internet can be a web of hope and possible remedies but it is also filled with traps, so be careful! Please don't part with your money easily – be prudent, there are people out there who are happy to sell you bogus products. Don't follow me down that road, instead join a group of fellow sufferers and carers, share remedies and help to support each other physically and psychologically. It is important to understand that because of the nature of Eczema, what may work for one person may be an allergen for another, or simply not work for you.

So we know that it's common and usual that products put directly on the skin respond for a while, then stop being effective so trust your instincts and follow them, enjoy the moments of successes, and learn from them all.

For example: the list of moisturisers we used are extensive. Sometimes the moisturiser would be fantastic instantly but would slowly become an irritant, other times the moisturiser would be an instant irritant. We found that moisturisers with a petroleum base were usually irritable for him. They would sit on the skin, rub off on everything and cause the skin to become hot. However we discovered that if we use them on top of creamy water based moisturisers they don't irritate. Other people swear that all petroleum based products are no good. However they have a place in our lives. Trust your instincts!

Our Lives Today...
...It wasn't all doom and gloom

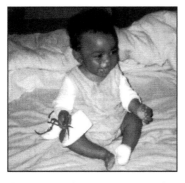 There were, of course times when Jayden was comfortable. We made the most of those times. He was a beautiful, handsome and intelligent child (he still is of course), and when he was comfortable he would dance and sing more often. He was talented, he would do things to make me laugh. What a gem! By the time he was 14 months old, Michael Jackson's 'Billie Jean' was his favourite song and party piece. He was so cute and expressive, he would sing the song and scrunch his face up as if he were feeling every word. We would sing and dance together almost every day, he was good at it and he loved it - he still loves to dance today.

By the time Jayden was five years old I could relax a little. Now in March 2014, he's 13 years old and life is very different from 2001. Jayden still has Eczema, food intolerances and Allergies, but it's less. It's easier to look after, because we are experienced. We both have a great understanding of his condition and Jayden does a lot to help in taking care of himself, so I'm no longer exhausted.

His Allergies are now down to seven things, we no longer have many unpleasant surprises, so we are happier.

Towards the end of Spring last year, Jayden developed a heavy rash over half of his face. By the end of the week it had spread all over his torso and arms. My prescription was for him to have a bath with a few drops of Tea Tree Oil every day, shower with Aveeno Body Wash, moisturise with Forever Living Aloe Vera Gelly to cool his skin; plus Aveeno Lotion. He drank 30mls of Forever Living Aloe Vera Juice each day and 2 liters of water. For the severe itching we dabbed on the pure Aloe Vera Juice and extra Gelly with Propolis Cream to the affected areas. He recovered from this flare up over a period of 3 weeks. We don't know what brought it on. We just take each incident as it comes.

His general daily routine is to wash in mild cleansers such as Aveeno Body Wash or Seba Med Face and Body Wash. For short periods of time he can use other non-specialist washes, however these are too harsh for him long term, but at times he just wants to, so he does. He moisturises often throughout the day: applying Coconut Oil, Aveeno Lotion then Neutrogena (Norwegian Formula) on top.

Some nights I still get interrupted because I hear my son scratching so I go to him to moisturise him and hold his hands away from his body until he settles. All this is done while he sleeps. A few nights a week the itching will wake him up as well, we go through the routine to cool him down and moisturise, however mostly he falls back to sleep quicker than when he was a baby. Thank God for that.

Jayden's condition hasn't prevented him from doing anything he's wanted to do. When he was four years old he started swimming lessons. I would have started him earlier but the Eczema was too severe. Today, he is an excellent swimmer and has reached Level 9 in his classes, additionally he's been scouted for a Swimming Club. The Chlorine can still be a problem so we have to ensure that he showers thoroughly and moisturises extra afterwards.

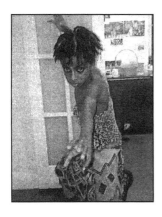

Jayden has always loved acting and when he was seven years old he joined The Anna Fiorentini Film and Theatre Saturday School. He has achieved some wonderful things since then. His greatest artistic achievements to date are playing Young Simba in the West End production of 'The Lion King' at the Lyceum in London; playing the part of Jerome in 'Rev', a television Sit Com, a number of short music videos and short films; he is a member of Zoo Nation Dance Company. In 2013 he played the character of Frankie in a 13 part series on CBBC, called Hank Zipzer. This Summer he records Series 2. He's living his life.

Jayden tells me he doesn't remember lots of the things I've written in this book and I'm happy about that. You can read his story on pages 151 - 156.

I have a theory that children who suffer greatly with medical conditions are very special indeed. Jayden is perfectly special and living proof of my theory.

Conclusion

Hindsight is beautiful

L ife would have been a lot easier had I known then what I know now, but they say everything happens for a reason, right?

I hope somehow the words in this book can help you, comfort you in some way and reassure you that things can be better and do get better.

Is Eczema a reaction to something or a lack of something? Is it a genetic predisposition that you have no control over?

Our GPs didn't have all the answers for us then and neither did I. Even today, thirteen years later, I have not found an answer to these questions. I can only conclude that it may be a combination of several factors? Many people swear by the effectiveness of Steroids and various other products, they swear by routines, medicines, doing this and not that. Who knows? I wanted to take you on our journey and share some of our experiences with you. I hope that your journey will be eased by what you have read.

Eczema is an allergy, it's an individual disease. Successful treatment for one person may be a complete failure for another. It takes time to get to know your child's condition and what worked today may not help tomorrow. Knowing this will help you to cope and not feel disappointed when products are no longer effective. You will see patterns in your child's health behaviour. Observe and take notes of what happens when this or that is eaten or touched. Make notes of different reactions in different environments and create a healing and learning atmosphere in your life.

Do your very best to follow your instincts, gut feeling, listening to the spirit, call it what you want, it's a powerful sense..., it works. On a number of occasions I felt insecure about the decisions I was making concerning my son because of the lack of 'clinical evidence'. But I had to do what the Professionals told me to do because I hadn't had this experience before, only to find out that I was right all along, however, it takes experience and confidence to trust your instincts. Having said this, Health Practitioners play a massive role in the care and treatment of illnesses and diseases and it's important that you work together so you can get the best outcome and feel empowered.

Today Jayden visits Guys and St Thomas's Hospital annually where he has Allergy Testing, Food Challenges and his Eczema is reviewed. The Consultants, Doctors and Nurses are amazing, helpful and understanding. They listen and respect all our concerns. We have since moved to Well Street Surgeries in Hackney and his GP's there are the best, they listen and we work together for the best possible outcome.

When I read through my diary I remember how helpless I felt...

...it didn't have to be like this.

Through the words I wrote, I can feel my desperation.

I know now that the Doctors, Consultants, Nurses and other Health Professionals were doing the best they could, they are not miracle workers. At the time I didn't think they were on my side and I wonder why I thought like that? Well the answer is that stress and lack of sleep can make everything more difficult. I felt the system was failing us, but in hindsight they did the best they could. I needed help with coping, but they do not have all the answers and neither do I.

The important thing to remember is not to blame yourself, or anyone else for that matter, when things don't go according to plan. Parents, Carers and Health Professionals all need to work together to do their best. Eczema and Allergies are so difficult to treat and to live with. As parents we can concentrate on our child/children and get a more thorough picture of them then the Health Practitioners because of the amount of time we spend with them, and the innate connection we have with them instinctively, so every effort should be made to make us feel respected, heard and reassured. Health Professionals have thousands of cases to deal with so they have great insight and experience into the disease, we should feel strengthened by this fact and together we can make a better life for sufferers.

For a long time I blamed myself for Jayden's suffering. I believed if I had followed a better diet during my pregnancy my son would not have developed Eczema or Allergies, however, I didn't know how I could have improved my diet to prevent this. Blaming myself didn't help me or my son. Coping with Eczema and Allergies is about getting support and by finding a group of fellow sufferers, you can discover so much more. As a group you feel reassured that you are not alone and that you can only do the best you can do.

I don't know 'WHY' Jayden and I had to go through all of this – but I needed to write our story down so you would know there is hope.

One of the many positive things that have come out of my son's condition is I became more interested in nutrition. I have studied it academically and now as a Health and Fitness Consultant I am able to help my clients on a deeper level. I understand the physical, emotional and physiological impact food can have on individuals and how it affects us all in different ways. I have my son to thank for that. I am also there to lend an ear and help where I can.

Thank you Jayden, my hero and my Champion.

Jayden's Story

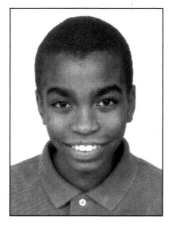

I do remember some of the stories my mum has written about, but not the really early days because I was too young.

I don't know how old I was but one of the things I really remember clearly is my Eczema making my nights endless and the unstoppably itching. Trust me, it wasn't nice. Some days I would itch so much that my skin would stick to the sheet, or I couldn't bend my knees because it was too painful, so I walked with my legs straight, just like a penguin. Sorry I'm not going to dumb it down, it is what it is, or shall I say 'it was what it was'! When I was scratching so much, one of the things that would stop me crying was 'Winnie the Pooh' videos. My favourite character was Tigger because he was funny and he cheered me up. He took my mind off my Eczema and made me happy. Even today I still love 'Winnie the Pooh'!

Another thing that took my mind off my Eczema was my mum's beautiful singing. Even now, when I'm really itchy it will calm me down and helps me to go to sleep.

My mum says that lots of nurseries said that I couldn't join then because of my Eczema and Allergies. They said it would be too much for them to cope with, can you believe that? I don't think that's right, do you? Nah!!!

A lot of people think that it's annoying to carry my medicine with me wherever I go, but to me, it's just the norm. It's just there, at the bottom of my bag and it's not a big deal, though sometimes it's pretty weird I have to have the the Epipens and Antihistamine in my bag ALL the time. It's quite cool at the same time because I've had to make little routines that will help me survive incase I come into contact with something I'm allergic to.

Having Eczema and Allergies is tiring sometimes as I have to always remember to moisturise my skin. Sometimes I have to do it over and over again because my skin just needs more, other times, it needs less. My mum is always saying, "Jayden, you need to put your cream on," and when I tell her that "I have", she says, "Go and put it on again then." We have lots of conversations like that, as you can probably imagine.

Some days I still get itchy, but I guess it's not that bad any more. I've just learned to cope with it, things could be worse. When my Eczema is good I feel like... well, like I don't have Eczema anymore. I can forget about it for a while, I feel comfortable and I can bend my hands without my skin splitting. When my Eczema is bad I hide my hands in gloves if I'm in a public place. I don't close my fists or things might get worse; I'll put lots of extra moisturisers on and just get on with it.

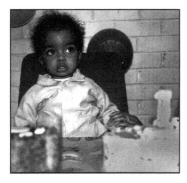 Other times it's really annoying having Allergies. At my first birthday party, yes I remember it, my mum thinks I don't – she says I just think I remember it because of the photos, but I really do! I was sitting there looking at everybody digging into MY cake, when I wasn't allowed it. I wasn't too happy, I just felt left out and really sad. And if you look at my face in the picture you can definitely tell that I wasn't a happy bunny. My mum says she made me a separate cake but I can't remember that bit.

Now, to make me feel better, my mum makes me chocolate bars or cakes. The chocolate bar my mum makes is really delicious – it has dairy free chocolate, nougat and... sorry, I can't tell you the secret ingredients! It's the best chocolate I know! Having my own cakes and chocolate bars made for me, makes me feel more special, oh and between you and me, I get to have more than everyone else!

My Allergies can become tricky when I go out to eat. It seems that too many restaurants don't know the impact food has on someone's body, they just look at food as something that should taste good and it doesn't matter what's in it.

For example, one day I went to a restaurant with my mum and I told the waiter what allergies I have because I needed to be sure that the food I was ordering was safe for me. He went and spoke to the chef and when he came back he said the chef would make sure that my food didn't contain anything I was allergic to. 'Alright' I said and waited for my food. When my food arrived it looked and smelt delicious.

Me and my mum began to eat. I must have taken two spoonfuls and my mouth began to itch. I told my mum I was having an allergic reaction so she got my medicine out. I didn't want to take it in the restaurant but she insisted I did – so I did. I was not happy about the mistake but kept it on the low and just asked mum if we could leave quietly, she wanted to complain and speak to the chef. I asked her not to – so she didn't. She asked the waiter to take the food away and told him what had happened. The waiter insisted that everything was done as we asked, he took no responsibility and he didn't even apologise. He even insisted we paid. I looked at my mum as if to say – please mum, just pay, I don't want a scene, I just want to get out of here. So she paid and we left quietly.

When we left I was upset and so was my mum. We talked about what had happened after the effects of the allergic reaction had gone and my mum made me a lovely dinner.

After having a reaction I don't like talking about it. My mum knows this and she gives me space. Having a reaction, especially in a public place makes me feel... odd, vulnerable, self-conscious, scared and angry because mostly it's because people just don't listen or understand how important it is that they listen to what I've said and avoid the ingredients I've told them I'm allergic to. It's simple!

Can you believe that I've been into restaurants and after I tell the waiter what my allergies are he says, '... it should be alright, it only has a little milk' or 'I don't know what the ingredients are but... it should be ok'. I mean they act like I'm the only one with allergies, like I'm some sort of alien!

These are not the only times that this has happened. Restaurants need to understand the implications of coming into contact with something you are allergic to. I don't understand what's so difficult.

It does feel quite uncomfortable that restaurants make such mistakes. It's very dangerous too. Things need to change so I wanted to talk about it and be part of that change.

Having Eczema and Allergies hasn't stopped me from getting on with my life. I'm now 13 years old and I love doing loads of things, but most of all acting, sing-ing, swimming, dancing, playing the drums, piano, steel pans and playing sports. When I was 9 years old, I spent 6 months playing Young Simba in 'The Lion King' at the Lyceum Theatre in the West End of London. It was magical.

I've done a few other acting roles and I really enjoy them. Last year year I was cast in a 13 part series called Hank Zipzer and this summer I'll be filming Series 2. It's been amazing, don't get me wrong I get turned down A.K.A 'rejections' from a lot of roles too and yeah, some-times I feel disappointed, but I'm quite happy that I'm being treated equally and not being discriminated against because of my Eczema and Allergies.

It just goes to show that you can achieve anything you desire if you put your mind to it, and lots of hard work of course.

References

On the next few pages, I have added my personal remedies, hints, tips and other useful information that I picked up along the way in our own battle against Eczema and Allergies.

I am happy to share them with you.

Please note that none of these are personal recommendations, please seek professional advice and make sure you find what is best for you.

Jayden's Allergies and Intolerances (Aged 3)

ALLERGIES/ UNTOUCHABLES	INTOLERANCES
• All nuts • Dairy products • Tomatoes • Strawberries • Lemons • Kiwi • Salmon • Trout • Eggs	• Soya • Fruits (especially banana and pear) • Salt • Lamb • Wheat • Hydrogenated fats • Processed foods • Artificial sweeteners and colours • Refined sugar • Oats • Newspaper ink • Latex • Rice • Potatoes

Jayden's Allergies and Intolerances (Aged 12)

ALLERGIES/ UNTOUCHABLES	INTOLERANCES
• Most nuts (not peanuts) • Dairy products • Kiwi fruit • Sesame seeds • Poppy seeds • Trout • Eggs	• Artificial sweetener & colouring • Bananas • Excess sugar • Excess salt

March 2013 and Jayden is no longer allergic to all nut (however we still avoid them); peanuts are perfectly fine, as well as lemons, strawberries and tomatoes. He has been given the all clear for salmon but doesn't like the taste much. His intolerances to wheat, rice, potatoes, salt and fruit have all gone. His body is more comfortable with artificial sweeteners, colours, processed foods and hydrogenated vegetable fats, however, we continue to avoid these as much as possible as they are not good for anyone's body!

Sugar is still an issue today – if he has it in excess, he becomes very itchy and the backs of his knees, hands and ankles flare up.

Allergy Testing

It's important to learn all about your child's condition and know what the triggers are. Get your child officially allergy tested as soon as possible.

Eventually, at almost two years old, Jayden was given a blood test which confirmed all the Allergies I had suspected. I knew the results all along but I was just relieved that the doctors would now believe me.

Scratch Test - this is done on both of Jayden's arms.

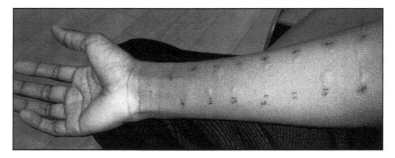

Today and over the last 8 years Jayden has the Scratch Test to check his Allergies at Guys and St Thomas's Hospital. This procedure determines allergic sensitivity to a variety of substances by applying them to scratches in the skin. I give Jayden £1 for every scratch, he came home with £23 the last time he had this done!

Bearing in mind, you might have to wait a long time for Allergy Testing, carry out your own food testing. The most effective way is to keep a diary so you can record what is happening to your child on a daily basis.

The intolerances can not be detected in the blood tests. Jayden's doctors continued to say that I should feed him the things I had eliminated as there was not enough evidence to prove otherwise. I ignored these requests because I had all the evidence I need-ed as there were many occasions when Jayden would have a reaction with different foods and products - I could clearly see the relationship. When he ate something sugary, two to six hours later he would have an itchy rash all over his body. He was intoler-ant to sugar. At first I couldn't work out what was happening, but eventually it all started to make sense. I know that if I was taking notes of his reactions in a much more constructive and detailed way, doing it as a planned observation and writing it all down from the beginning, I would have come to my conclusions much earlier.

LET MY HINDSIGHT BE YOUR KNOWLEDGE.

Personal Remedies and Tips

Trigger factors and precautions:

Do seek professional advice.

- **Allergens** - Be aware that certain foods may cause flare-ups. Allergies can be caused by anything, some common ones include: eggs, cow's milk, peanuts, soybeans, fish, or hot and spicy foods and some less common ones such as: seafood, sesame seed, soy and wheat.

- **Animals** - Be aware that playing with animals may cause Eczema flare-ups. Some children with Eczema are allergic to cats, dogs and other furry animals. Be observant and before introducing a pet to the home, arrange for your child to spend time with it outside the house to ensure that there are no negative reactions.

- **Chemicals** - Stay away from products that irritate the skin like harsh soaps, perfumes, bleach or detergents when washing clothes or bedding etc.

- **Cool environments** - Eczema skins are generally hot and therefore not happy in hot, dry environments. In a hot environment Jayden will itch more, especially if the environment is also dry. However, when we visit warm climates, we always stay by the beach and we've found that the combination of sun and sea is healing. As long as he is kept cool at bedtime, he thrives in the sun. You can keep a room cool by leaving windows open or using a fan, leaving a bowl of water in the room to keep some moisture in the atmosphere is also helpful.

- **Cool products** - Cool your creams, moisturisers and emollients in the fridge before applying as this will further help to calm hot skin.

- **Emotional stress** - One of the most difficult trigger factors to predict in children is emotional stress. Children with Eczema often react to stress by experiencing red itchy rashes and flushing. For a child with Eczema, normal feelings like anger, frustration, and fear can lead to an Eczema flare-up. Allow your child to be expressive. Try to make your child's environment as calm and happy as possible, no matter how stressful you get in the course of treating them.

- **Establish a routine** - Knowing what order you do things in will take the pressure off when things flare up – for example, bath with emollient, pat dry, oil skin whilst damp, apply lotion, apply cream, put on bandages, feed, read a story, put to bed. Of course you need to remain flexible because sometimes you may just need to do things differently to satisfy the need.

- **Humidity** - Monitor humidity. Low humidity can dry the skin, especially on cold winter days. High humidity and heat can lead to increased sweating and make the itching worse – balance is key.

- **Find a babysitter/accept help** - Get a network of family and friends to relieve you from childcare. It's essential that you get a break from the constant role of caring. It's all too easy to forget about yourself when caring, so I would recommend finding a babysitter you can trust and making time to go out with friends, have a day or an hour to yourself, re-ignite your hobbies, or anything else you want to do for rest and relaxation.

- **Join a support group -** Caring for a child with severe Eczema and Allergies is a full time job and you can begin to think you are the only one in the world going through your battle. Meeting fellow carers is a great support as you can share ideas and listen to each other – simply being together can take the desperation away.

- **Keep a diary -** If you write about your day noting routines and incidences, you may well discover a pattern or trigger for good and bad times, thereby avoiding the bad and increasing the good.

- **Lots of water (hydration)** - The body is made up of 70% water - keep hydrated to help the body keep in tip top working order. Give your child the amount of water they need and monitor that they are also urinating enough.

- **Nutrition -** Good nutrition has a major role in our wellbeing – after all, we are said to be 'what we eat'. Helping your child's body to be strong and healthy by putting great nutrients into it will ensure the body can be at its best. It goes without saying that you should avoid all the foods that the child is allergic to and by keeping a diary you'll know what he/she thrives on. Eating foods as near to their natural state as possible and having a balance is a good guide for good nutrition thereby arming your immune system to fight. Get advice from a professional nutritionist.

- **Saliva** - A common problem for young children with Eczema is that their own saliva is often an irritant, which is why their cheeks and the skin around their mouths can often be affected. Applying a barrier cream was helpful for Jayden.

- **Scratchy fabrics** - Avoid wool or other scratchy fabrics. Choose breathable fabrics - soft fleeces in winter and cool, smooth cottons in summer are the best choices we found.

- **Sleep, rest, relax and have fun!** - I cannot stress enough the importance of physical rest, emotional relaxation and actual fun. It is far too easy to become over- 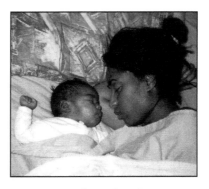 whelmed with your situation and only focus on that, I was guilty of that for some time. Stress can negatively affect your baby and you will not be able to cope as well if you stay that way. Making time for sleep, rest, relaxation and fun are extremely important. Focus on doing fun activities and ensure that you and your child have a lot to laugh about, this helps to relieve the stress thereby alleviating the symptoms. Your relationship with your child is more than their condition. Sleep.

Remember you can only do the best you can do. Take one day at a time, or break it down even more and take one moment at a time. Don't beat yourself up.

- **Temperature** - Ensure your child does not get over-heated. After active play periods, dab sweat away with a damp cloth, pat dry, keep their bedroom cool and bed covers to a minimum.

Products That Were Helpful

- **Aloe Vera - Forever Living** - Eczema is an inflammatory disease and Aloe Vera helps reduce inflammation. My son drinks this daily and I have been known to dab it on his skin when he's very uncomfortable as it gives him some relief, helps to speed up healing, is packed with nutrients and assists in boosting the immune system.

- **Camomile - dried flowers** - The calming effects of drinking this tea is well documented, it can also be added to the bath and used directly on the skin to soothe irritation.

- **Evening Primrose Oil -** This is a great internal moisturiser to be taken long-term. I used the oil in capsule form by popping it open and squeezing it into Jayden's mouth when he was two years old. I also massaged it on very dry areas of his body (but only at night as the smell is strong). As Jayden got older he would chew the capsule until the oil seeped out. Today he'll just swallow the capsules.

- **Lavender Essential Oil -** The health benefits of Lavender Essential Oil include helping to induce relaxation and relieve pain. It's a natural disinfectant, it enhances blood circulation and helps respiratory problems. I use a few drops in his bath or as an infusion.

- **Seba Med Face and Body Wash** - Ph balanced and gentle on the skin.

- **Tea Tree Oil** - Tea Tree Oil has a long history of positive, traditional uses. Australian Aboriginals use Tea Tree leaves for healing the skin: taking care of cuts, burns and infections. I found that a few drops in Jayden's bath helped with his mild skin infections and keeps them at bay today.

- **Udo's Oil** - This is a wonderful blend of Omega Oils 3, 6 and 9, (essential fatty oils) which Jayden would take as a food supplement.

Moisturisers

For all the products that I've listed, ask your GP about them. He/she should be happy to look them up if they are unfamiliar. My GP hadn't heard of using Propolis in the treatment of Eczema, he looked it up then prescribed it for Jayden.

The list of moisturisers we used is extensive and the benefits vary. Sometimes moisturisers would be fantastic instantly but quickly become an irritant, other times an instant irritant and sometimes great for ages.

We went through dozens of moisturisers. Below are just a few which helped:

- **Aveeno Products -** Johnson & Johnson Ltd

  My son is using Aveeno Body Lotion, Aveeno Cream and Aveeno Bath Wash. This is our latest break-through, he has been using these for over two years and he is still comfortable with them. The full range of Aveeno products can be found online at www.aveeno.com. You can get some of these products on prescription. Speak to your GP if you're interested in trying them.

- **Avène Products**

The products produced at Avène Spa were very helpful for Jayden. At Avène we used the water continuously to drink and bathe in. In London we use the Avène water spray in the canister. The Cold Creme was very soothing and moisturising for a time and today we use it on and off. There are many Avène skin care products – you can go to their website and check them out. Avène staff and the products produced there really understand Eczema. You can purchase these through the internet and at large chemists. www.avenecenter.com

- **Aloe Propolis Creme** - Forever Living

You can get other brands of Propolis Cream from your GP. This product is helpful on infected skin and speeds up healing. It's a heavy moisturiser which I apply to the thickened parts of his skin. I would use this after rubbing it in my hands to warm it up and thin it out a little, I then add something oily on top such as Liquid Paraffin/soft white paraffin or Norwegian formula, available from your GP. It has a very strong smell so we only use it at night or if he's staying at home.

- **Chickweed Cream**

We purchased this from The London Clinic of Phytotherapy, my son really loved this cream. Students would sit in on our consultations and prescribe under guidance. I would pay a very reasonable rate plus the cost of the prescription. Each session lasted 45 minutes – this was great value for money. It was the best moisturiser to date. Later this organisation moved and I couldn't find them anywhere. We found variations of the Chickweed Cream but nothing as good as theirs. We continue with their other recommendations of Lavender and Camomile.

- **Olive Oil**

This was recommended as the purest moisturiser and I used it when Jayden was 1 week old. Initially we purchased the one they sell in the chemist produced for skin applications however, it seemed to make my son's skin even drier. I have since been told that it was because Jayden's skin was so dry that the olive oil had this effect. Dry skin pulls it right down into the skin layers. The advice was to keep putting it on until the skin healed (in other words, no longer dry). I admit I didn't persevere to this extent.

In the early days I would add a little olive oil with whatever cream he was using. Jayden said it made him itch and he didn't like the smell. However, I have always added it to his food.

Today we use Extra Virgin Olive Oil on his skin and in his food. It doesn't leave a smell and is very hydrating. Shop around and see which one you like.

- **Petroleum Based Moisturisers**

We found that emollients with a petroleum base were usually irritable for Jayden if we used them directly on his skin. These emollients sit on the skin, rub off on everything and can cause the skin to become hot. However, I find they have a place in his treatment - we put these moisturisers on top of other water based moisturisers and they help to keep the skin moisturised for longer by locking the moisture in.

- **Shea Butter**

I would purchase this from an African produce shop: it was a block of pure Shea Butter which resembled a roughly put together bar of soap wrapped in cling film. I was advised that this was not hygienic and I shouldn't use it. However, I didn't have a problem with it. I tried the other Shea Butter products in a jar, but they were not as effective, they were full of additives and perfume and proved to be a very poor substitute – the more 'hygienic and acceptable' brands irritated Jayden's skin!

This block Shea Butter is a fantastic product on my son's skin. I rub the moisturiser in my hands until it melts and then apply it to his skin. This makes his skin feel supple and comfortable. When Jayden was little he loved to play with it. I would put a small lump of it in his hand and he'd squash it until it melted. I didn't like the strong smell it had, but because it was the most effective moisturiser he had to date, we used it for a few months, then it simply didn't work anymore, instead it made his skin hot and itchy. I stop using it for a while and then go back for short periods of time. It's very helpful.

Other creams we used:

- DOUBLEBASE Moisturising Gel
- Cetraben Bath Wash
- Oilatum Bath Additive
- E45 Moisturisers and Bath Additives
- Aveeno Bath Oil
- 50/50
- Vaseline
- Neutrogena - Norwegian Formula
- Organic Coconut Oil

Tips for applying moisturisers:

- Spoon your moisturisers out of the container so they do not become contaminated by you constantly going into the jar.

- Smooth moisturisers in a downwards direction so that the hairs are smoothed flat, thereby creating less likelihood of irritation, therefore less itching, which leads to less scratching.

Organisations Offering Help

The following organisations were useful for us:

- **Applejacks Health Shop, London**

  I spent many desperate moments in this shop. The Assistants are helpful, caring and knowledgeable; whatever they don't know they will quickly find out.
  Address: 28 The Mall, Stratford, London E15 1XD
  Telephone: (+44) 20 8519 5809
  Fax: (+44) 20 8519 1099
  Email: robert@applejacks.co.uk
  Website: www.applejacks.co.uk

- **Avène Health Spa, France**

  Marie-Ange Martincic (Director)
  Telephone: (+33) 4 67 23 41 87
  Website: www.avènecenter.com
  Website: www.avènehydrotherapycenter.com

Getting Avène treatment on the NHS

The following information is taken from the NHS website and outlines how to secure NHS funding to be treated at the Avène Hydrotherapy Centre:

"People with Eczema and psoriasis who want to visit Avène for treatment should ask their GP to refer them to a Dermatological Consultant who will recommend them for treatment to the Primary Care Trust. They also need to get an E112 form from their local post office to apply for funding (this covers a set period of medical treatment only and excludes travel or accommodation costs)."

- **Eczema Parents Circle**

  This is an online support group for parents of children with Eczema. The group invite you to their 'circle' to share your experiences of caring for your child with Eczema and creates a place to express how Eczema has affected you as a parent, as well as listen to others sharing their emotions and experiences.

- **Eczema Voice**

  This is a site for people with Eczema. It offers a newsletter, helpline, discussion board, hints, tips and remedies.
  Website: www.eczemavoice.com

- **The Haywards Heath & District Eczema Support Group**

This is a voluntary group set up by people with first-hand experience of Eczema. They are unable to give specific medical advice, but have regular meetings which give people with Eczema and their carers a chance to exchange ideas or simply have someone listen.
Website: www.communigate.co.uk/sussex/eczema

- **National Eczema Society**

The National Eczema Society has two principal aims: first, to provide people with independent and practical advice about treating and managing Eczema; second, to raise awareness of the needs of those with Eczema among Healthcare Professionals, teachers and the government. It's very informative.
Telephone: 0800 089 1122
Website: www.eczema.org

- **Skinship - founded by Ashley Medicks**

This is an independent organisation set up to help people suffering with skin diseases. Ashley can lend a reassuring ear and welcomes calls from anyone with any kinds of skin problems. There is no website, however, you can find extensive information about Skinship if you search his name on the internet.

- **Talk Eczema**

An online community support magazine founded by a mother whose daughter suffered from the chronic condition. The content here is clear and helpful.
Website www.talkeczema.com

Two parents share their stories

A Typical Tale

Terri Scott and her daughter Ruby

My daughter Ruby is four years old. She has had Eczema since birth. It was always 'manageable' to an extent, meaning no soaps, certain dietary requirements and moisturisers which would need to be put on about five times a day. Itching, sleepless nights, red eyes and eyelids and looking unwell were normal for Ruby. Whenever her skin got irritated this would cause a 'flare up' which always meant a trip to the doctors and them prescribing a steroid to put on the affected red areas. No other advice or options are given.

The end of summer 2010 should have been a great time for Ruby because she was getting ready to start school but this was actually the worst time ever because of her skin. She had a massive flare up with her skin turning red and blotchy from head to toe. She would scratch all day and night, even though her skin was bleeding and coming off in front of our eyes. This affected her sleep a lot which meant she was miserable and cried a lot – this was how she started school.

Needless to say, I went to the doctors and they sent us to the children's skin department at Homerton Hospital in East London. When we were seen, I explained the situation and how it was affecting our lives, expecting more

support than I normally get at the doctors. Straighta-
way the doctor looked at Ruby's skin and said, "She needs
to be covered all over in steroids for two weeks and she
needs to have medicine to help her sleep at night." I was
shocked and very upset. I explained I didn't want to keep
on covering the problem with Steriods, I wanted it to
go away; I wanted to find the root of what irritates the
Eczema so it can stop. I was bluntly told there is no "miracle cure" for Eczema, it's just a matter of getting on top
of it and dealing with it. The doctor was insensitive and
added, "What do you want me to tell you?"I left the hospital in tears and felt so helpless for my baby girl.

The real shock came later on when I read the information
from the medicine prescribed for sleeping and itching –
it is also used as a sedative for children having minor
operations. I never used the medicine because I didn't
feel right about it, but, I did use the steroid to calm
the irritation and since then another new moisturiser and things seem to be getting better for now. This
whole experience has left me feeling that the support and
treatment for Eczema is very poor. This is not right
and things need to change.

Sarah Furness and her son Gene

2 July 1998 - 1am, awake and tired. My beautiful boy unsettled scratching at his legs and hands.

From diary: A difficult week!

I'm so tired all the time. I am awake, unable to sleep, it's 1am and I have had to get up. We share a bedroom when you become unsettled, like tonight, and I can hear you scratching. I have managed to settle you a little. I have come out of the bedroom to get a drink and try to relax. I need to sleep but cannot. I can hear you scratch and whimper in your sleep. Last week we were at the hospital to see the doctor about your skin which is sore and inflamed with infection at the moment.

My feeling of helplessness is immense; your hands are red and swollen, cracked and infected. The infection hits so quickly once your hands become cracked, the infection takes over in just a couple of days.

You are just starting to talk and this is brilliant and so hard at the same time. You lift your little hands to me and say "sore" with tears in your big blue eyes. What can I do to take the pain and discomfort away? Very little. Your skin looks so raw, it is raw and bleeding. During the nights you scratch so hard you looked as if you'd break your fingers you put so much pressure into scratching and rubbing your hands, wrist and legs.

The sound of you scratching keeps me awake, you don't get a good night's sleep and there is blood on your bedding in the morning. You look up from your cot, hands held high with blood on PJ's, looking tired, you say "sore mummy, hands sore". What can I do, I bath you, love you, wrap you in bandages, but I cannot take away the constant discomfort you feel. They send men to the Moon, but they can't treat you and take your pain away. I am now hypersensitive to the sound of scratching. I tense up and feel tearful at the sound of anyone scratching at work or on the tube. The sound of scratching on fabric makes me jump.

You are on your 3rd course of antibiotics in a row, we have to bathe you in this pink stuff called potassium – you seem to be on the mend now. Your hands are the worst I have seen them. You bend your fingers and they crack and bleed. You still manage to smile and laugh even though you can't hold your spoon or a pencil properly. You can't climb the climbing frames at the park because your hands crack and bleed. But you manage to run around and laugh. At the library at story time, some woman removed her child from playing near you and asked me if you were infectious and could pass it on. I suppose it's perfectly natural to try and protect your child, but I was torn up by her action. Your hands are so cracked and infected, with blood and puss. It feels so unfair.

Our routine is to apply Fucibet on your hands and Eumovate on your legs twice a day. I hope that all the steroids doesn't harm or scar your skin. Given all this it still seems to bother me more than it does you.

Diary: 2012 - my beautiful boy is now 6'3" and 16 years old.

Where have all the years gone? Today my son has very little Eczema, mostly just dry hands and some reoccurring spots on his legs. He now manages this himself and amazingly the whole ordeal of bandaging, infections he cannot remember. He cannot remember waking at night crying because his hands were sore. He is amazingly good natured and continues to bring joy and pleasure. The experiences of early life with Eczema almost seems another lifetime away.

Bibliography & References

- Dr H M Ramsay – Consultant Dermatologist and Honorary Senior Clinical Lecturer. Department of Dermatology, Royal Hallamshire Hospital

- National Eczema Society

- Skinship Helpline - Ashley Medicks

- Coping with Eczema, Dr Robert Youngson. Sheldon Press. 1995

- Avène Health Spa – France

- Allergy Magazine. 'What's the Alternative' Jan-Feb 2004 pg 85)

- Robert Dobson, Mail Online 'Rain can lower Eczema Risk'

- The Low-Salt Water Study, The Pierre Fabre Institute Dupuy P, Cassé M, André F, Dhivert-Donnadieu H, Pinton J and Hernandez-Pion C. (1999)

Websites

- www.applejacks.co.uk
- www.aveeno.com
- www.avènecenter.com
- www.babycenter.com
- www.breastfeeding-problems.com
- www.diaryofadesperatemother.com
- www.eczema.org
- www.eczemavoice.com
- www.communigate.co.uk/sussex/eczema
- http://groups.yahoo.com/group/
- eczemaparentscircle/info
- www.medicalnewstoday.com
- www.medicinenet.com
- www.molnlyckehealthcare.com
- www.netdoctor.co.uk
- www.nhs.uk/livewell/allergies/pages/foodallergy.asqx
- www.talkeczema.com

Glossary

- **Allergy** - A food allergy is a rapid and potentially serious response to a food that doesn't bother most other people. It can trigger classic allergy symptoms by your immune system (see Anaphylactic shock). It's an adverse, hypersensitive disorder of the immune system.

- **Allergy Testing** - This measures the level of allergic reaction to a variety of substances. With this information an action plan can be devised so that the patient doesn't come into contact with the allergen.

- **Anaphylactic Shock** - This is a severe allergic reaction that can be triggered by a food allergy, drug, or an insect bite etc. A severe reaction of this type can include the following symptoms: itching of the skin, a raised rash (like a nettle rash), swelling of the lips, tongue, throat, hands and feet, flushing, weak pulse, tightening of the chest, difficulty in breathing, fall in blood pressure and in some cases loss of consciousness. In this case an Epipen will be needed until further, medical help arrives.

- **Antibiotics** - The word antibiotic comes from the Greek word 'anti' meaning 'against', and 'bios' meaning 'life'. Antibiotics are also known as anti-bacterials, they are drugs used to treat infections caused by bacteria. Bacteria are tiny organisms that can sometimes cause illness to humans and animals.

- **Antihistamine** - In allergic reactions, special allergy cells in the body release chemicals called Histamine. Histamine causes rashes, sneezing, itching, swelling and other allergic reactions. Antihistamines stop the Histamine from working in the body, by reversing the reaction the allergen caused.

  Histamine can cause more serious, sometimes life-threatening reactions such as Anaphylaxis as the person goes into Anaphylactic Shock.

- **Cannula** - is a hollow surgical needle used to create a temporary entry to a vein or artery so that drugs can be given intravenously to a patient at any time without having to repeatedly puncture the patient's skin.

- **Epipen (pronounced 'a-pip-en')** - This is a single dose medicine (injection kit) of Epinephrine which is administered to counteract a severe allergic reaction until medical help arrives. It is an Adrenaline that tries to counteract the body's reaction to an allergen.

- **Hives** - also known as Urticaria, Welts or Nettle Rash. It is a raised, itchy rash that appears on the skin. The rash can be limited to one part of the body or spread across large areas of the body.

  The affected area of skin will typically change within 24 hours, and usually the rash will settle within a few days. If it clears completely within six weeks, it is known as acute urticaria. (NHS Choice. www.nhs.uk/conditions/nettle-rash/pages/introduction.aspx

- **Intolerances** - are more common than allergies. Symptoms come on more slowly often after many hours after contact. Symptoms can be rashes, bloating, cramps and itching etc.

- **Naturopathy** - as a form of alternative medicine based on a belief that a special energy called 'vital energy' or 'vital force' guides bodily functions. Naturopathic philosophy favours a holistic approach and seeks to find the least invasive measures necessary for symptom improvement or resolution, thus encouraging minimal use of surgery and unnecessary drugs. According to the Association of Accredited Naturopathic Medical Colleges, "Naturopathic medicine is defined by principles rather than by methods or modalities. Above all, it honours the body's innate wisdom to heal."

- **Patch Test -** this is a way of identifying whether a substance that comes into contact with the skin is causing inflammation. The substance is applied to the skin and observed over a few days for a reaction.

- **Rickets -**is a deficiency disease resulting from a lack of Vitamin D, typically from insufficient exposure from sunlight. In children it can be characterised by defective bone growth, it can also affect general health. You can find Vitamin D naturally in fish, fish liver oil, egg yolk and a number of breakfast cereals and other food products which are fortified with it. It is essential for strong bones because it helps the body to absorb calcium and a variety of other vitamins and minerals from the diet.

- **Scratch Test -** this procedure determines allergic sensitivity to a variety of substances by applying them to scratches in the skin.

- **Topical Steroids -** are used to suppress the inflammation in the skin. They have no effect on the underlying cause of the inflammation, but they do control the flare-ups and can help to relieve symptoms such as itching and redness.

- **Tubifast -** garments are ready made garments for use in dressing retention and wet or dry wrapping. www.molnlycke.com

- **Vallegan -** typically, used for sedation for children from the age of 3, unless prescribed by a Doctor for younger children. Can also be used for hives.

- **Ventouse -** is a contraption that sucks onto the top of a baby's head like a plunger and helps with the labour by pulling baby out.